The Longevity Key

Published in the UK in 2024 by

Copyright © Dr Rob Shepherd 2024

Dr Rob Shepherd has asserted their right under the Copyright, Designs and Patents Act, 1988, to be identified as the author of this work.

All rights reserved. No part of this book may be reproduced, stored in a retrieved system or transmitted, in any form or by any means, electronic, mechanical, scanning, photocopying, recording or otherwise, without the prior permission of the author and publisher.

Paperback ISBN: 978-1-7385542-0-1
Hardback ISBN: 978-1-7385542-2-5
eBook ISBN: 978-1-7385542-1-8

Cover design and typeset by Spiffing Publishing

The Longevity Key

Dr Rob Shepherd

FRCP, FRCP (Edin), FRCP (Glas)

Contents

Introduction 7

Chapter 1
    Healthspan and Biological Age 10

Chapter 2
    Genetics 16

Chapter 3
    Comments of Two Centenarians 29

Chapter 4
    Longevity Historically 33

Chapter 5
    Historic Brutal Killers 38

Chapter 6
    Effects of War 48

Chapter 7
    Three Phases of Medicine 57

Chapter 8
    Mediterranean Diet 63

Chapter 9
    Important Features for Longevity 66

Chapter 10
    Cure Obesity 72

Chapter 11
    Intermittent Fasting 80

Chapter 12
    Some Foods to Avoid 85

Chapter 13
    Antioxidants 93

Chapter 14
    Sleep and Stress Reduction 110

Chapter 15
    Exercise and Walking 119

Chapter 16
    Drinking Water 130

Chapter 17
    High Blood Glucose – Diabetes 132

Chapter 18
    Ultra-Processed Foods 136

Chapter 19
> Benefits of Coffee 143

Chapter 20
> Bread... 147

Chapter 21
> Bananas, Lemons, and Broccoli 149

Chapter 22
> Turmeric 153

Chapter 23
> Conclusion.. 155

INTRODUCTION

Who is this book written for and why did I write it? Throughout my life with 45 years as a Consultant Physician, I have been interested in diagnoses and have tried to help people generally. I am recently retired and with my breadth of knowledge and recent significant research, I think I can give some very useful advice and information – which will help the individual person to live longer and hopefully in better health. My specific interest in longevity started about seven years ago when I read a very interesting article in the Sunday Times which discussed a village in the French Pyrenees near the Spanish border. This village has the greatest longevity in Europe and the men can live up to 115 years old and are healthy. They have no coronary heart disease, no strokes, and no vascular disease. This is followed by the second-longest longevity hotspot in Sardinia. Both these places have "a common denominator" which I will discuss in the section on red wine. This longevity contrasts with the UK where men live to 79 and women to 82.9 (according to 2018-20 statistics).

The book is written to indicate what you need to do to live longer. Basically, there are 10 things to do – see chapter "Important Features for Longevity". Interestingly only the other month, some newspapers got hold of a paper from the

US which described eight features, one being avoidance of drug addiction. Embellishments in the book include deaths due to major illnesses, wars, etc. If your main aim is to gain information about your health you may decide to skip those chapters and concentrate on chapters marked with an asterisk* referring to the contents page at the front of the book.

This book is meant for the benefit of the general public – and is not the read for geneticists or high technology scientists. I do discuss some scientific evidence and some biological/genetic mechanisms where appropriate – but I am trying to make it an easy read so the average person can understand and follow the advice given if they wish.

If you buy a new car (and I am a car enthusiast) you will be proud and it should be perfect. Even if it is an Aston, Porsche, or Lamborghini, if you do not maintain it then it will develop problems. Likewise, if we do not look after/maintain our bodies, the body will deteriorate and we will age more rapidly and have a reduced lifespan. As we get older, we tend to have more body damage and the repair systems get weaker.

IMPEDIMENTS TO LIFESPAN

Smoking reduces your life expectancy by 10 years and in a smoker, "the big four" factors are:
1. Diseases of atherosclerosis (ageing vessels)
    - cardiovascular disease
    - cerebrovascular disease (stroke)
2. Cancer

3. Neurodegenerative diseases and dementia
   - Parkinson's
   - Alzheimer
   - Vascular dementia
   - Lewy Body dementia
4. Insulin resistance

Insulin Resistance is not a disease per se but is basically a metabolic condition which occurs in a range of conditions from non-alcohol fatty liver disease (NAFLD) to type 2 diabetes. It is clearly important and, under normal circumstances, as it is not a disease it would not appear on a death certificate.

By trying to reduce "the big four factors" one would have a great benefit on longevity. So if you stop smoking, drink red wine in moderation, have a healthy diet, exercise, and get good sleep you may well avoid coronary artery disease.

CHAPTER 1

HEALTHSPAN AND BIOLOGICAL AGE

Most people would like to live to an old age (achieve longevity) but importantly want to remain mobile, healthy, and not confused (i.e. no dementia). In other words, apart from longevity, they really want good healthspan ... a comparatively new term coming from the US referring to good health throughout life even in old age. In the UK, you will recall that the current lifespan is 79 for men and 82.9 for women (based on 2018–20 statistics).

The problem is if you develop certain diseases, particularly as you get older, healthy living is affected and your healthspan is reduced. It is interesting to note that when I qualified as a doctor (MB, ChB) in 1968, we were taught that the diagnosis was all important – and in my early years, there was usually one diagnosis to concentrate on and possibly two or three others that were not important at the time. Previous illnesses were usually under previous history (PH) in the notes. At the end of the consultation, a triangle would be written (signifying diagnosis), and if there was a differential diagnosis, two triangles would be written. For example, in the case of chest pain, the differential might be listed:

1. Ischaemic Heart disease
2. Hiatus Hernia
3. Musculoskeletal Pain

This was at a stage when those over 65 were considered elderly and were of retirement age, and if they lived to their mid-70s, they were 'doing well' and those in their 80s and 90s were an exception. The UK's current state pension age is 66. These demographics worldwide are an increasingly ageing population. In 2023 in France, the retirement age was raised from 62 to 64 with a requirement that the retiree had worked at least 43 years. The three countries with the highest retirement age of 67 are Iceland, Norway, and Israel. On the flipside, Saudi Arabia has the current lowest retirement age at 47.

Then as the years went on, and the population lived much longer, it became apparent that in many cases patients would have multiple diagnoses. This became apparent to me when I became Senior Medical Registrar in Radcliffe Infirmary, Oxford, and quite often there might be eight to ten total diagnoses on the list … with perhaps the first two being most relevant to the admission. Amazing how times have changed! Soon after becoming a Consultant Physician (1976), I remember one professor sending a request that all letters should have a list of diagnoses at the beginning of the letter. This seemed very sensible and made management much easier for general practitioners when they subsequently saw the patient and indeed helped hospital doctors if the patient was later seen in the clinic. Over the years the number of diagnoses seems to have increased further and sometimes patients are on as many as 15 or

20 medications. In general, polypharmacy is not the ideal situation and so often I have tried to reduce the number of tablets taken – you have to recall drug interactions and side effects … and the decision-making can be difficult.

HEALTHY OLD AGE (HEALTHSPAN)

Healthy old age can be affected by almost any medical condition, some more seriously. If you have chest pain due to angina then life can become unpleasant and you may have therapy with nitrates (GTN and beta blockers (Bisoprolol). If the function of the left ventricle is affected you might get breathless on exertion or on lying flat (orthopnoea) then you may continue diuretics, but the left ventricular (LV) function can be improved by the addition of an ace-inhibitor such as Rampiril or possibly Spironolactone. The latter is not advisable if there is impaired kidney function as it can cause a rise in potassium. There was a phase many years ago when it was popular to do coronary artery bypass grafts (CABG), which are vein grafts taken from the legs and used to bypass the arterial narrowing in the heart. At that stage in my life, as Registrar of the National Heart Hospital London, I helped with the post-operative cases of Donald Ross, who did the first heart transplant in the UK, and Magdi Yacoub, a famous heart surgeon of worldwide renown. Nowadays, CABGs are largely superseded by stents, the areas of narrowing having been ascertained by arteriographic studies (coronary arteriogram). These usually stop the angina symptoms but we need to recall the basic disease process. So it is better not to have the disease in the first place. You should not smoke, have no sugar, eat healthily, and do some exercise – features which I discuss elsewhere in this book.

If you are arthritic, for example, rheumatoid arthritis or osteoarthritis (OA), joint pain can be a problem which affects happy and healthy living. Mobility may become seriously impaired and there are several medications available – perhaps the most common being non-steroidal anti-inflammatory agents such as ibuprofen. If you have bad OA hips or knees then life can become very unpleasant, with sometimes greatly reduced mobility, and one of the options may be surgery. Within the NHS there is a waiting list and when you have distress and an uncomfortable lifestyle, then life is not particularly happy.

DIABETES MELLITUS is a very significant medical diagnosis as it can lead to so many complications over the years. If well controlled you may escape with no problems – but so many systems can be involved. The worst are cardiovascular and cerebrovascular disease problems – which include angina and heart attacks (myocardial infarction with its damage to heart muscle). These are related to blood vessel damage and in the case of the brain, there can be transient ischaemic attacks (TIAs) or actual strokes (cerebral infarctions). Peripheral blood vessel damage in the legs can cause pain in the calf or if on walking (intermittent claudication) or with vessel occlusion or critical blood supply gangrene may occur, with necrosis of tissue. This may be just in the toes going blue and ulcerated, and later may go black and perhaps shrivelled up. Alternatively, the whole foot may be involved and the foot may become offensive and smelly. The cases have to be carefully assessed. If there is just pain while walking it may be possible to do arterial bypass surgery but if there is very extensive gangrene peripherally, an above-knee amputation might have to be considered. Many of these scenarios can be prevented. You must not smoke ... or if you are a smoker, give up. Clearly, diet is important, avoid sugar at all costs – and read my discussion on red wine (later chapter).

BIOLOGICAL AGE

Biological age is the rate at which you are ageing physically and can differ from your chronological age. There are some centres in the world where specific parameters can be looked at in the laboratory and biological age determined. If you are a smoker you have a more advanced biological age and your lifespan is 10 years less. If you look young for your age then in all probability, you have a younger biological age.

Professor David Sinclair, an eminent geneticist at Harvard University, has measured his biological age. He is now about 52 and considers his biological age, based on scientific information, to be about 10 years younger. He looks young for his years and has adopted four habits:
1. Eats a plant-based diet
2. Intermittent fasting
3. Reducing stress
4. Regular exercise

Personally, I adopt the latter three, all of which I consider very important. Probably I am a bit down on leafy vegetables as I am not really a salad person. Another feature in my book is to have plenty of antioxidants – including red wine, walnuts, blueberries (which I sprinkle on my porridge each morning), raspberries, and strawberries.

DO WE LOOK YOUNGER?

If the answer is "yes" then we are younger biologically. At present, we cannot measure a person's age biologically or genetically, but scientists can now look at a DNA methylating clock, reading the chemicals that indicate age, and that information can be matched with how old someone looks with an Artificial Intelligence (AI) technique – i.e., AI interpretation of age. In summary, if someone looks older then they are truly older in general.

CHAPTER 2

GENETICS

Many people think that your longevity is down to your genes. Well, this is partly right – 20% of longevity is due to the genes, but 80% of health in old age is how you live your life – and if you are healthy you turn on the longevity genes. The human body is incredible. When we are born we have 96 billion cells and 23,000–24,000 genes. There are 50 genes for longevity and these regenerate cells and make proteins which tell the body what to do.

GENOME

All the DNA of an organism is called a genome. Some genomes are small such as those found in bacteria and viruses, but some genomes can be very large as found in some plants. DNA is a polymer, a large and complex molecule, which is made up of monomers called nucleotides. Interestingly, the human genome has about 3 billion nucleotides – cf. one Japanese flower with 150 billion nucleotides.

DNA, as you will recall from your school days, is made up of two linked strands that wind around each other to form a twisted ladder – a shape called a double helix, as discovered by Watson and Crick. Each strand has a backbone made up of alternating sugar (deoxyribose) and phosphate groups. Attached to each sugar is one of four bases – ATCG: adenine (A), thymine (T), cytosine (C), and guanine (G). The two strands are connected by chemical bonds between the bases:

adenine – thiamine
cytosine - guanine

The sequence of the bases (nucleotides) along the DNA backbone encodes the biological information such as instructions for making a protein or RNA molecule.

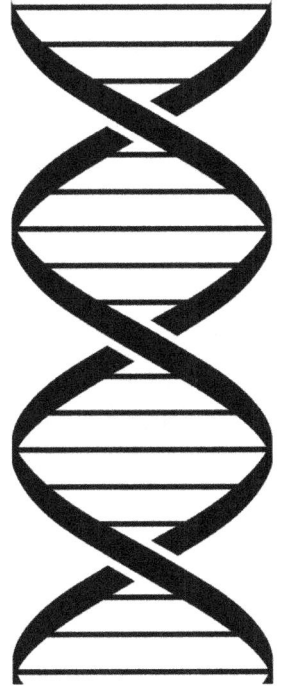

"Double helix"
(The solid line is the sugar-phosphate backbone)

The DNA is mainly in the nucleus but some is in the mitochondria.

HALLMARKS OF AGEING include:

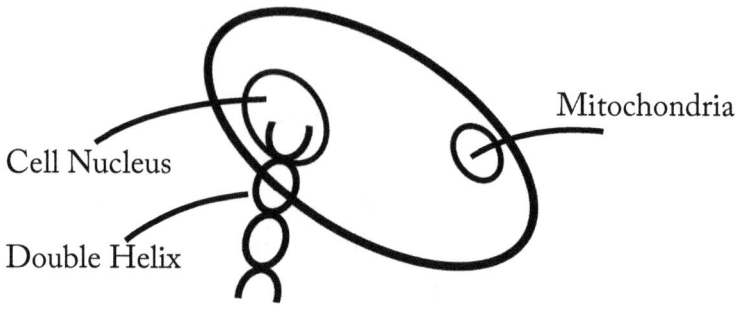

1. Telomeres
2. Sirtuins and mTOR
3. Mitochondria
4. Stem cells

TELOMERES

You will recall from your school days the word "telomeres", the long bits of chromosomes. They get shorter with age. When we are young the repair system is good but as we age the repair system gets complacent and the telomeres get shortened.

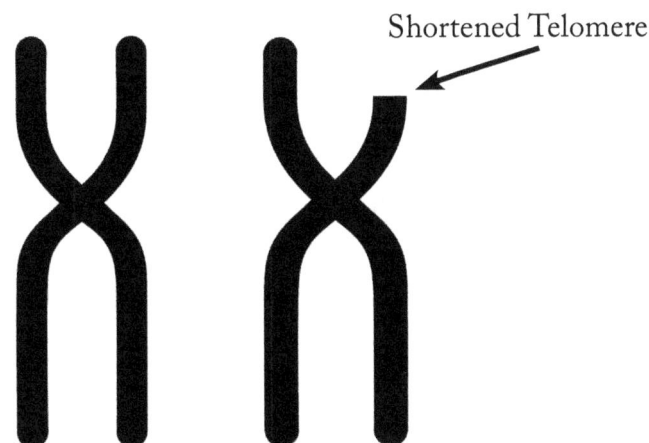

Telomeres

Interestingly, a study in mice in which the telomeres were lengthened with telomerase was associated with increased longevity by 40%. You might think this is the answer but the snag is the treatment may cause pre-cancer cells to develop and proliferate.

Stress impacts the length of telomeres, by the release of glucocorticoids – which enter the cells and cause a cascade of damage. If there is stress early in life it tends to persist throughout life. For example, children subjected to violence have shorter telomeres. Clinically, mothers of ill children – and therefore they have had to deal with a lot of stress – have shortened telomeres and are 10 years older in terms of their telomere length.

Management of stress leads to increased telomerase activity in red blood cells – thereby increasing telomerase length. Interestingly exercise gives the elderly longer telomeres, particularly if they do sports and have moderate or vigorous exercise regimes – by exercise I mean walking up and down stairs, gardening, volleyball, and aerobics. Vigorous activities include running, cycling, tennis, gymnastics, and jumping. To have this benefit it needs to be done at least three times per week.

Diet also has an impact on our telomeres. We get longer telomeres with fruit, dairy products, meats, and legumes. Interestingly the consumption of coffee is also associated with longer telomeres.

SIRTUINS

You may not have heard of the term. In fact, there are seven of them (SIRT1 to 7). They are enzymes that use nicotinamide adenine dinucleotide (NAD) to remove acetyl groups from proteins. Without getting too involved in the science, they slow ageing and basically repair things. If there is not enough protein to make the sirtuins then we age more rapidly. So if there is a broken chromosome, and therefore a risk of cancer, we need the sirtuins to chip at the repair on the chromosome. If there is inadequate protein then the sirtuin can not be made and the repair will not occur. Professor David Sinclair, the eminent geneticist at Harvard, has aptly likened their activity to being "little Pac-men" or "like Jack the Builder chipping away at the defect and doing repair". Sirtuins are like scissors chipping acetyl off a protein. The older we get the sirtuins become less active and the spool of DNA, rather like a garden hose around a pole, gets looser.

Proper lifestyle and physical activity increase the level of sirtuins, and it is thought that this increases the lifespan. It is SIRT-1 and SIRT-3 which are affected by fasting and have an effect on insulin response and oxidative effect. Some have suggested they may also have an anti-cancer effect.

Sirtuins require NAD and the accelerator on them is Resveratrol. This is a polyphenolic compound which occurs in red wine which was the stimulus to my research and writing this book. Resveratrol occurs naturally in the skin of red grapes, walnuts, peanuts, and some other plants. It has been shown to have anti-ageing benefits. With Resveratrol activating sirtuins, it is worth noting it increases SIRT-1 eightfold – and this leads to faster DNA repair, weight management, and lower inflammation. There are studies which prove that resveratrol (anti-oxidant) becomes active with running, gardening, gym exercise, and fasting – the sirtuins are turned on and make more DNA. So with this mechanism it is all beginning to tie in together ... red wine, walnuts, strawberries, raspberries ... and exercise and fasting (particularly intermittent fasting) – each of which is discussed in later sections of the book.

In animals, there are three pathways that affect longevity – sirtuins, mTOR and AMBK. All are affected by hunger – and it is thought the same principle applies to humans. So intermittent fasting (described elsewhere in the book) would fit in with all this. In a 2005 paper (Sinclair at Harvard), it was documented that one sirtuin gene was activated in animals by eating less. This boosted the level of mTOR and protected against DNA damage.

Loss of function of SIRT-1 is implicated in several pathological processes such as endothelial dysfunction (lining of coronary arteries), atherosclerosis (hardening of arteries and fat deposition), cardiovascular disease, hypercholesterolaemia (raised cholesterol), hypertension, diabetes, and obesity.

In one mouse study at Harvard University, one group were given a 25% reduction in calorie intake while the other group starved one day and were allowed free eating on the next. This had the same longevity benefit as the mouse that was on a greatly reduced calorie intake. So the take-home message, by extrapolation, is that probably we can have some fasting and then good eating – and have greater longevity.

mTOR GENE.

You probably will not have heard of this gene, which acts as a central regulator of cell metabolism, growth, proliferation, and survival. When you eat protein the mTOR gene is activated. It is responsible for regulating protein production and therefore directly influences cell growth, division and survival. If you eat a lot of protein, as in a steak meal, you will activate mTOR and if you have a lot of protein you will put on a lot of muscle. We certainly need muscle growth, particularly as we age, and a certain degree of muscle mass is important for longevity. You would think all this is good but too much mTOR is linked to age-related diseases like diabetes and cancer.

If you reduce/down-regulate the activity of mTOR you have greater longevity. This is because of "autophagy", which basically is the recycling of proteins. If the protein is in short supply then to make a new protein, the gene will recycle the old protein, which is very advantageous. Reduced mTOR activity occurs with stressful situations, such as those produced by intermittent fasting – which is discussed later in the book. If one eats a lot of meat, the mTOR will not attack the old protein and this builds up. Increased mTOR activity is seen with tumour formation, insulin resistance (type 2 diabetes), and obesity.

We need to consider bodybuilders. Weight-lifting is good for increasing muscle bulk and it increases the male hormones and makes people feel good. Bodybuilders often lift weights for 60–90 minutes per day, and they often take meat and protein supplements. You need more protein to sustain activity and to build up muscle. It is also important for the average person as they get older. Activating mTOR plays an important role in building up muscle. This increase in mTOR is all right in the short term but in the long term, the mTOR needs to be reduced/down-regulated to achieve longevity. The answer to this is to give the body a periodic break from processing the amino acids leucine, isoleucine, and valine, and this break allows for a reduction in mTOR and helps longevity. In other words, at that stage, we are inducing stress (hormesis) and this leads to mTOR reduction and stimulation of mitochondria through the stress (mitohormesis).

So the take-home message is that it is important to keep a balance. The increased mTOR leads to muscle growth, which in short bursts is good and healthy, for the average individual and bodybuilders. But if that happened all the time with high mTOR, that situation is linked to a shortened lifespan, cancers, and many chronic health conditions. So the solution is to have occasional high-protein meals and then go for intermittent fasting which will reduce the mTOR and help longevity. We have to note that too little mTOR can lead to health issues with muscle atrophy and delayed healing.

AMPK ACTIVATION

AMPK is Adenosine Monophosphate Protein Kinase which is an enzyme which is the body's regulator of energy metabolism. I am discussing this because of its critically important action in making more mitochondria which have been described as "the powerhouse of the body". The mitochondria are important for metabolising what we eat and making chemical energy. Poor mitochondrial function is associated with heart disease, type 2 diabetes, insulin resistance, metabolic syndrome, and dementia.

AMPK is closely linked to blood sugar. When the body is fasting and starved of glucose (as in fasting) the AMPK is activated. Some scientists have noted that Metformin, a drug used to treat type 2 diabetes, can lower the level of glucose, enhance insulin sensitivity, and reduce symptoms of ageing. Further research is being done in this area.

MITOCHONDRIA

Mitochondria are essentially ancient structures and lie outside the cell nucleus. These structures are the powerhouse of the body and they significantly determine – or are a major factor – in longevity. The mitochondrial theory of ageing suggests that an accumulation of damage to the mitochondria as you age may be associated with oxidative stress.

"Choose your parents wisely" is a comment I would like

to discuss. As a young medical undergraduate at Liverpool University, I was in a medical firm at Liverpool Royal Infirmary. Every Friday, we had the Friday Class, where a row of eminent consultants sat on the front row and a medical student would present a clinical case and be grilled on the information by the consultants. On one occasion I remember Dr Baker-Bates, an eminent Rodney Street physician, going on stage and conversing with a particular student, saying, "Well, my boy, it is important to choose your parents wisely." I thought the comment bizarre and regarded the physician as "different". In those days he was thought to have manic episodes and in today's terminology, he would be described as bipolar. The incident stuck in my mind and I realised it was partly true as genetics plays some part in longevity. At that stage, I did not know how much it contributed to old age but we now know that genetics are responsible for 20% of longevity. We now know that all your mitochondrial DNA – the powerhouse of the body – comes from your mother. So it is important to look at the female line of inheritance. Ideally, you want good lineage on your mother's side.

I will discuss an example. I told a pal of mine in Norfolk that I was writing this book and I started to mention genetics and longevity. He said, "Well I should be all right then as my dad lived to 82 and Granddad (on father's side) lived to 93." I went on to explain that 80% of longevity is related to how you live and 20% is due to genetics. A lot of people think if parents or grandparents lived to a ripe old age then they will probably do likewise. In my Norfolk pal's case, the longevity on the male side is not relevant. You want good genes on the female side. With this in mind, for clarity, I would like to discuss the Royal Family tree and some sections of my own family tree.

ROYAL FAMILY TREE

With the accepted fact that all mitochondrial DNA comes from the mother, we need to look at Queen Elizabeth II who lived to 96. Her mother, who for most of my life was Queen Elizabeth The Queen Mother and wife of King George VI, was a Bowes-Lyon and lived to 101.

So looking at the Queen Mother's Bowes-Lyon family tree, we note that her mother died at age 75, which was perhaps a reasonable age in 1938. I do not know the cause of death but remember in that era antibiotics were not available and could cause havoc. Clearly, Queen Elizabeth the Queen Mother had exceptionally good genes and passed these on to her daughter, later Queen Elizabeth II.

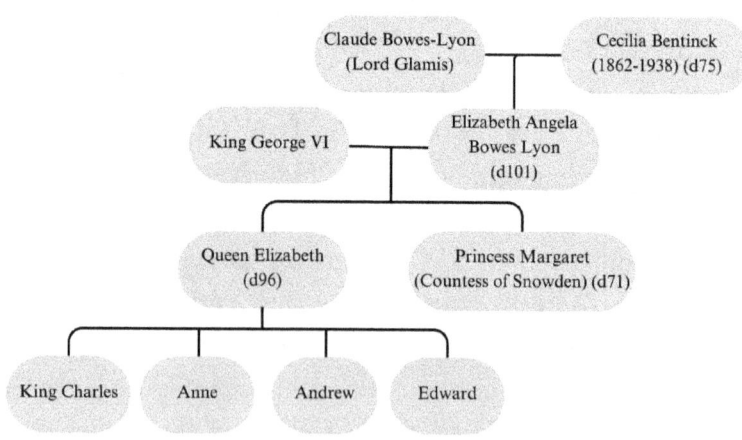

However her other daughter, Princess Margaret, only lived to 71. She inherited good genes too but one might consider she had a rather fast life but more importantly, was a smoker. A few years before her death, she had a lung operation and apparently, she had a total of three strokes (cerebrovascular accidents), the last one being the cause of death. Clearly, smoking was the factor that affected her cardiovascular system and caused her to live a much shorter period than her sister, Queen Elizabeth II. So the children of Queen Elizabeth – Charles (King Charles II), Ann (Princess Royal), Andrew (Duke of York) and Edward (Duke of Edinburgh) – will all have good genes and would be expected to have significant longevity and reach a ripe old age. But remember this has to be kept in perspective as 80% of longevity is dependent upon how we live. As regards the children of King Charles, their longevity genetically would relate to the Spencer family tree, as Lady Diana was a Spencer. So William (Prince of Wales) and Harry (Duke of Sussex) will carry none of Queen Elizabeth II's genes.

MY OWN (SHEPHERD) FAMILY TREE

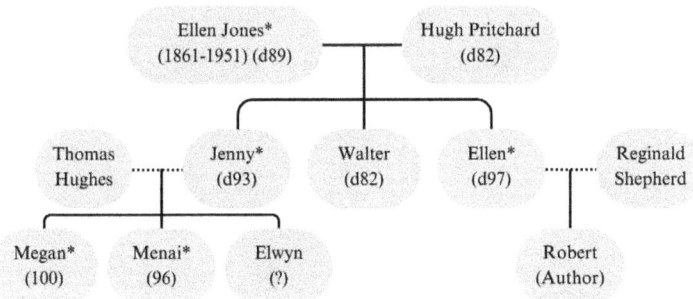

In my family tree, I would particularly like you to look at the female line – the various names marked with an asterisk*. My grandmother, Ellen Pritchard (nee Jones), died in 1951 at the age of 89 – which was considered a remarkable age at that time. She had two daughters (Jenny and Ellen) who lived to 93 and 97, and a son who lived to 82. That son was a sm oker so that would have reduced his life expectancy by 10 years and he had a lot of stress in his life (for example, in WWII he was in a landing craft in Walcheren Raid in Holland and six doctors in that boat were killed).

As regards Jenny's children, one son died aged 85 but had medical issues for years. It is important to look at the daughters now 96 and 100. So the critical thing about all this is the inheritance of the mitochondrial DNA. Clearly, Ellen Jones had excellent DNA and this explains the longevity of Jenny (my aunt) and Ellen (my mother). Jenny passed the good DNA on to her children and I should have my mother's DNA. My agent for medical work in latter years thinks I might hit "the ton"… and am hoping so if I keep up a good lifestyle.

CHAPTER 3

COMMENTS OF TWO CENTENARIANS

COMMENT OF A CENTENARIAN

Nowadays a number of people live to 100 or older, but it is uncommon for men to live to that age. According to a New England Centenarian Study based in Boston, Massachusetts, among the Centenarians 85% are women and 15% are men.

In April 2023, Today.com in the US reported that Vincent Dronsfield of Little Falls, New Jersey, was 109 years of age. His story is interesting and I will quote his comments. Dronsfield says he is lucky and enjoys healthy longevity. His routine is to go to town each day, buy his lunch in a restaurant and shop for groceries. He lives alone, his wife having died 20 years ago, and his children and grandchildren call. His recipe for a long life is spending time doing what you love. He worked until the age of 60 as an auto parts manager and in his late 70s, he retired as his wife said it was time to quit work. He served 80 years in the local Fire Department and he thought this social contact with friends helped him enormously. He also said he has a good sense of humour and he thought that helpful.

His recipe for a long life is:

1. Spend time doing what you love
2. Always keep moving – and by this, he was referring to walking and not sitting down a lot. He did not lift weights or do gym activities
3. He says to eat what you enjoy – and he takes Italian food, hamburgers, salad and milk chocolate. He drinks coffee each day and an occasional beer.
4. Good social contact with family and friends

WHAT IS MY TAKE ON ALL THIS?

Clearly, social contact is very important – in his case the Fire Service and family contact. It is important to do what you enjoy and I myself keep a lot of interests going, including gardening and landscaping, general running of the home, photography, films, news, and particularly international travel. I note that Dronsfield did daily visits to town and I myself am eight miles out of town so tend to do the shopping about twice a week.

A very important point, not mentioned by him, is to be motivated. I tend to give myself daily tasks ... and I must admit I get disappointed when I do not achieve what I set out to do. A workman who visited me to carry out some work said, "I presume you have a full-time gardener." I duly explained that it was me! It certainly keeps me busy. Dronsfield said he always keeps moving and I think this is a very important feature. I think it is critical because it helps one to stay slim (burning up calories), helps general mobility, and helps prevent coronary artery disease. One workman said to me that going up and down stairs in my house (three stories) will give me a lot of exercise.

Remember man was a hunter-gatherer and was always racing about to get food or avoid the sabre-toothed tiger. We need exercise and were not designed to be couch potatoes spending hours in front of the television or stuck on the internet. I remember in my job as a Consultant Physician I did a fair amount of desk work naturally but a lot of the time I was on foot, walking about on ward rounds and latterly going around the ward with a team using a Computer on Wheels. Even in the clinic one would be up and down from the desk to examine the patient on a couch. Dronsfield stressed exercise but did not lift weights or go to the gym. I must say I think this helps keep the muscle strength as we get older, and I have a pull-up bar between my bedroom and bathroom, keep a couple of weights handy, and actually have a gym in the cellar.

I have a bone to pick with Dronfield's diet. I do not consider hamburgers a healthy option – but we have to remember that he is American and they are almost a staple food there. But they are not healthy. I must not be too critical as my butcher does excellent sausages and I have to admit I occasionally deviate from my current white meat/fish main course and have three sausages for lunch. This regime is fairly new for me, since writing this book, as previously I enjoyed steaks and lamb chops particularly. I certainly think the chicken/fish regime is much more healthy. In one recent hotel abroad I went for the very healthy option and was having smoked salmon after my porridge at breakfast time and as hors d'oeuvre sometimes at dinner. Certainly, fast foods are to be avoided from a healthy eating viewpoint but on two occasions I was starving, once in Sydney and believe it or not in Moscow, and was so pleased to find a McDonalds!

I note Dronfield likes to take chocolate – and I refer to eating chocolate later in the book. Dark chocolate with 85% cocoa is the best.

ANOTHER CENTENARIAN

I was very interested today (Dec 2023) to read on GB News about a retired physician, now aged 102, and she explained her diet and longevity features. Apparently, this retired physician practised till the age of 88 and her recommendations included:
1. Drink lots of water
2. Get your vegetables as fresh as you can
3. Use meat that agrees with you
4. Avoid what does not work for you
5. Have a strong sense of purpose
6. Don't stop moving

What is my take on all this? Firstly, nothing was particularly made of the fact that she continued working to an advanced age. I think this means she was motivated and enjoyed her job, and she herself listed "a strong sense of purpose". This is clearly important – having a major interest. I continued in active Consultant Physician work until aged 76, which was indeed interesting on a day-to-day basis. Maybe the general public retire too soon.

I must suggest her advice to drink plenty of water is very important as is the comment, "Don't stop moving". I certainly subscribe to both of these concepts.

CHAPTER 4
LONGEVITY HISTORICALLY

According to anthropologists' examination of 5000-year-old skeletons, people lived to 40 years old in the Bronze Age. In the time of the Roman Empire 2000 years ago, the usual life expectancy was 30–45 years. Some well-to-do Romans however, lived to the age of 70. Over the years life expectancy has increased and in the UK, Europe, and the US, life expectancy is currently about 80 years. It is roughly static but there was a slight reduction following COVID. It is worth looking at longevity throughout history:

Ancient Egyptians	19–34
Romans	30–45
England 1600	24.7
1700	49.4
Early 1900s	55
1950	Under 70
2018–20	79 (m) and 82.9 (f)

ANCIENT EGYPT

Ancient Egypt had a very high infant mortality rate due to infection and the average age of death was 19 years. A lot of early deaths significantly skew the average lifespan and that can give the wrong impression. A mathematician would easily understand that and I had to think about the concept. So if the individual survived early age, then the age of death was 34 years for men and 30 for women.

ROMAN TIMES

In Roman times (2000 years ago), the life expectancy is often quoted as 30–45 years with deaths due to birth complications, sickness, poor diet, and wild animals. But one has to recall the overall figure is skewed by the infant mortality rate. A review of records as far as possible suggests that if you made it to adulthood and were a wealthy, educated citizen you would be expected to live to your 70s.

ANCIENT CHINA

In ancient China the population was small and life expectancy was 22–35 years. Marriage occurred early – for example, in the Ching Dynasty 16 for men and 14 for women. The mortality was high. Their more recent longevity is similar to that of Europe:
1850   32 years
1965   44.5 years
1980   65.5 years
2020   76.6 years

UNITED STATES

In the US, the expected lifespan is 76.4 (2022). In 2021 the three leading causes of death were heart disease, cancer, and COVID-19 – followed by diabetes and kidney disease. Information from the Centre for Disease Control (CDC) indicated that the deaths from COVID-19 and drug overdoses, most notably synthetic opioids like Fentanyl, caused a drop in life expectancy. Deaths due to liver disease or cirrhosis caused by alcohol, and deaths by suicide, shortened the lifespan. One has to note that the majority of these deaths are in younger people – and this significantly skews the life expectancy figures. In other words, a death at 20 affects the figures greatly, compared to a death at 75.

AFRICA

In Africa let us consider Lesotho (formerly Basutoland) and Nigeria. Lesotho has the lowest life expectancy in the world at 55 years for men and 56 years for women, and Nigeria has the lowest life expectancy for women at 54 years.

CARIBBEAN AND LATIN AMERICA

In the Caribbean and Latin America in 2021 the average life expectancy for men was 73 and 79 for women.

Barbados has the highest-ranking life expectancy in the Caribbean with 77.6 years for men and 79 years for women. This is because Barbadians have a good quality of life with good health care – the Queen Elizabeth Hospital provides acute care in a wide array of medical specialities. There is also access to food, disease control, and sanitation.

The leading cause of death in Barbados is dengue fever and the last outbreak was in 2016. It is a mosquito-borne disease. When I first retired, I spent six months out there on the West Coast (only to return to my UK home and start doing locum consultant work) and I well remember two delightful neighbours who were almost paranoid about mosquitos. They had an interesting machine with some blue lights which used to buzz and fry the mosquitoes. I used the air conditioning and kept the doors and windows shut. I remember my gardener taking me to the home of one of his US customers who had a front-line property on the beach and I noted the large open-plan dining area. It was interesting to hear that the multi-millionaire owner had recently been very ill with dengue. It made me think the open-plan dining in the evenings would significantly increase the risk. As I have said dengue is mosquito-borne and the Ministry of Health prioritises fogging exercises. I well remember being in my house and hearing unusual noises. On looking out, I saw tremendous clouds of fog down the road and immediately closed the open patio doors. I knew nothing about this and later learned what had been going on. I was so pleased I did not have open-plan dining like the guy on the coast.

Relating to mortality overall out there it is worth noting the infant mortality in 1960 was 69.6 per 1000 and by 2018 was 11.8 per 1000. This is a great improvement but it is still above the 4 per 1000 in developed countries.

SAN MARINO, MONACO, and HONG KONG

San Marino and wealthy Monaco have the longest life expectancy (2022) and Hong Kong is not far behind.

San Marino   85 (m) and 89 (f)
Monaco   84 (m) and 88 (f)
Hong Kong   85.2

JAPAN

Japan has a life expectancy of 82 years for men and 88 years for women. The low morbidity is attributed to a low rate of obesity, low consumption of red meat, and high consumption of fish and plant foods such as soya beans and tea.

CHAPTER 5
HISTORIC BRUTAL KILLERS

The diseases that spread across international borders and reaped havoc, leading to the greatest deaths in history are:
1. Black Death (1334–53 – Bubonic plague (75 million–200 million)
2. Cholera (1853–54) – 23,000 deaths in GB
3. Smallpox – more than 300 million since 1500
4. HIV/AIDS

BLACK DEATH

The Black Death was a bubonic plague epidemic due to Yersinia Pestis and was spread by the bite of infected rat fleas. It caused 75 million–200 million deaths between 1334 and 1353. This was the greatest cause ever of death from infectious diseases. It hit Europe in 1348 and reached England in June of that year. Interestingly it probably started in Crimea, where Phoenician traders were involved, and spread to Europe. It came to England by flea-ridden rats in boats and fleas on the bodies and clothes of sailors.

Over the next two years (1348–50), the disease killed between 30–40% of the population. The pre-plague population of England was 5 million–6 million so there were about 2 million deaths in England. The total number of deaths in Europe (including England) over that period was 25 million–30 million.

The incubation period of bubonic plague was two to eight days and people developed sudden high fever, headaches, chills, muscle aches, weakness, and one or more swollen glands (called buboes) – hence the name Bubonic Plague. Nowadays, plague can be successfully treated with antibiotics.

CHOLERA

Cholera is acquired by drinking water or eating food contaminated with cholera bacteria (Vibrio Cholerae). About 1.3 million–4 million around the world get cholera each year and 21,000–143,000 die from it. Four major outbreaks occurred in London between 1832 and 1866 and led to the deaths of tens of thousands of people. It causes severe diarrhoea and dehydration. As well as diarrhoea, there is vomiting, leg cramps, and feeling weak.

The first cholera pandemic occurred in the Bengal region of India near Calcutta (now Kolkata) in 1817–24. The disease dispersed from India to Southeast Asia, the Middle East, and East Africa through trade routes. It reached Europe in 1830 and the first epidemic in Britain was in 1832 when 52,000 died. From 1853 to 1854, the epidemic in London claimed over 10,000 lives and there were 23,000 deaths for the whole of Great Britain. Dr. John Snow conducted an investigation into the cholera epidemic in London and he demonstrated that contaminated water was the main source of the epidemic. The 1854 outbreak was stopped by John Snow convincing a London local council to remove the handle from the Broad Street pump in Soho. The cholera epidemic in the neighbourhood came to an abrupt end. John Snow could not convince other doctors and scientists that cholera was spread when people drank contaminated water until a mother washed her baby's nappy in a town well in 1854 and kicked off an epidemic that killed 616 people.

It is worth recalling that in the mid-1800s it was thought that cholera was air-borne from rotting organic matter, and was particularly prevalent in the slums with overcrowding. It turned out that it is a water-borne disease caused by contaminated water sources. In the mid-1800s London's poorest areas were affected by contaminated water and other filth, as basement cesspits overflowed due to the lack of an efficient sewage system. The Thames, the main source of drinking water for residents, became more and more polluted.

In London the need to clean up the Thames was irrefutable. There was a terrible stench coming from the Thames during the hot summer of 1858. It was so bad that it drove MPs out of Parliament. In June of that year Disraeli, the eminent Victorian Prime Minister, tabled The Metropolitan Local Management Amendment Bill, and within 18 days a bill was created, passed, and signed into Law for the refurbishment of the entirety of the River Thames. It just shows what can be done and should be a lesson for today's politicians!

SMALLPOX

Smallpox is due to the variola virus and is one of history's deadliest diseases. It produces a pustular skin eruption and during that stage, there is a general spread of the virus throughout the body (viraemia), which causes local lesions in the pharynx (back of the throat), tongue, larynx and trachea (airways), and oesophagus (pipe to the stomach). It also caused potential lethal chest complications – interstitial pneumonitis (a type of pneumonia).

As I have said, it is one of history's deadliest diseases – with more than 300 million deaths from this since 1500. However, the history of smallpox may go back to 10,000 BC at the time of the first agricultural settlements in northeast Africa. It seems probable that it spread from there to India through ancient Egyptian merchants. The earliest evidence of skin lesions resembling smallpox is found on the faces of mummies from the time of the 18th and 20th Egyptian dynasties. The mummified head of pharaoh Ramses V (died 1156 BC) bears evidence of the disease. At the same time, cases in China were described and ancient Indian Sanskrit texts refer to the condition. I have only recently learned, on doing more research, that the first stages of the decline of the Roman Empire (AD 108) coincided with a large-scale epidemic. This is known as the plague of Antonine and may well have been smallpox.

In the Middle Ages, smallpox was a very significant disease and in those who contracted it, the mortality was 20–60%. We have to note the Spanish and Portuguese conquistadors going to the New World and introducing new infections to a population with no immunity to the new bugs. It is thought smallpox was introduced in this way. The disease decimated the local population and was instrumental in the fall of the Aztec and Inca empires. Similarly, the disease was introduced to the eastern seaboard of North America by the new settlers and this led to a decline in the native population. Another fact to consider is the slave trade which we have heard a lot about in recent years. However, I have only just come across the fact that the slaves came from parts of Africa where smallpox was endemic. I had not heard about that in my history lessons.

In the 18th century, it was referred to as "the speckled monster" with a rash appearing suddenly and those who survived had disfiguring scars. In the whole of Europe throughout that century, there were 60 million deaths – which works out to 400,000 each year. This figure included five reigning monarchs.

In the UK up to the 19th century, smallpox is thought to have accounted for more deaths than any other infectious disease, even plague and cholera. In the City of London, more than 320,000 people are recorded to have died from smallpox since 1664.

In school, I learned about the Franco-Prussian War of 1870–75 but there was no mention of smallpox at that particular time. For the younger generation, this was a war between Prussia (later part of Germany) and France. When I was researching smallpox I found out that vaccination was mandatory in the Prussian army so you would expect the Prussian state to be protected from infection. But the French soldiers were not vaccinated and there were small outbreaks of smallpox in the French prisoners of war. This then spread to the Prussian population (now part of Germany) and to other parts of Europe.

Variolation is the intentional inoculation of an individual with smallpox material, and this dates back to 16th-century China. Usually, there is the injection of liquid, found inside the pustule of a smallpox individual, under the skin of a healthy person. This would usually result in a milder infection of smallpox after which the person is immune against the disease.

Variolation was introduced in Europe by aristocrat Lady Mary Wortley Montague in 1717. She observed the practice in the Ottoman Empire (currently Turkey) when her husband was the British Ambassador in Istanbul. She pushed the Government for Government Mandated variolation in England. In 1722 the two daughters of the Prince of Wales were inoculated. Thereafter, variolation became a practice in Great Britain and became known in other European countries. In France, King Louis XV died of smallpox in 1776 and his successor and grandson, Louis XVI, was inoculated with the variola virus one month later.

Around this time (1716), it was brought to public attention in the American Colonies that enslaved West Africans had long practised this technique. In this year, Cotton Mather was told about this practice by his slave Onesimus and Mather publicised this and argued for its use in the Massachusetts smallpox outbreak of 1721.

EDWARD JENNER (1749–1823), a physician in Gloucestershire, pioneered the first-ever vaccine against an infectious disease. He had been inoculated with smallpox at the age of eight and later as a physician, variolation was part of his work. In 1796 he heard a milkmaid say that having cowpox made her immune to smallpox and this caused him to think about the subject carefully. He noted that milkmaids who had had cowpox were protected from smallpox. He observed that people who had suffered from cowpox would subsequently have a very mild if at all, visible reaction to smallpox inoculation. He hypothesised that inoculation (variolation) using the cowpox virus would protect children against smallpox as well.

In May 1796, Jenner inoculated a boy called Phipps with cowpox. He felt unwell for several days but made a full recovery. Two months later he took matter from a smallpox sore and inoculated Phipps with it. Phipps remained in perfect health and was the first person to be vaccinated against smallpox. His research had met with a lot of opposition, including the Royal Society, but he published an increasing number of cases. His new procedure was referred to as a vaccination. There had been some reservations but by 1801 it was considered safe.

Even the President of the US, Thomas Jefferson, was impressed and in 1806 wrote to Jenner – included in that letter is the comment,

"You have erased from the calendar of human afflictions one of its greatest."

Certainly from 1800, the number of smallpox deaths declined. Mandatory smallpox vaccination came into effect in Britain. In due course, Britain had the Vaccination Act of 1853 which made it compulsory for all children born after 1 August 1853 to be vaccinated against smallpox during the first three months of life. In 1959, the World Health Organisation (WHO) passed a resolution to eradicate smallpox globally – but funding was insufficient to meet global needs, with consequential vaccine shortage.

1918 FLU EPIDEMIC

The 1918–19 flu epidemic caused 16 million deaths, more than the deaths in World War I. It was a deadly influenza pandemic caused by the HN1 influenza A virus. It started like any other influenza virus, with a sore throat, chills, and fever. Then the virus ravaged the patient's lungs – leading to respiratory failure. Autopsies showed hard red lungs drenched in fluid. I was told a story about my uncle who worked throughout the epidemic in Royal Navy Hospital, Haslar, Portsmouth – the main Naval hospital in the UK. The Navy sailors all presented with typical flu-like symptoms but then the vicious twist occurred, with an attack on the lungs. Within hours the sailor often turned cyanosed (bluish-black), due to poor oxygen supply. When the feet became black they were carted off to die. My uncle was on the frontline and saw numerous sailors die in this fashion.

The virus probably originated in Fort Riley, Kansas, in March 1918. There was overcrowding and insanitary conditions which led to the propagation of the virus and within a week, 522 men were admitted with severe influenza. Similar outbreaks occurred in Virginia, South Carolina, Georgia, Florida, and California. It seemed to affect the military personnel and not civilians. By May 1918, influenza began to subside in the US. Soldiers at Fort Riley, now ready for battle, were shipped across the Atlantic but were incubating the virus in the long cramped voyage. Then on arrival in France, the symptoms appeared with "three-day fever" or "purple death". Soon the French had purulent bronchitis, the Italians called it Sand Fly fever and the Germans called it Flanders Fever. They all presented the same symptoms my uncle had witnessed. In the US it affected many personnel docked at east coast ports with patients suffering from influenza and pneumonia.

The flu occurred in three waves. The first wave started in March 1918 and soon spread throughout Western Europe. Then in the summer a more lethal type developed – striking fast and vigorously. Some victims died within hours of their first symptom, others in a few days. Post mortem showed lungs full of blood and these poor servicemen really suffered. The epidemic generally became a pandemic – and within four months it spread around the world. The second and third waves occurred in the winter of 1918.

Interestingly, young adults who were usually unaffected by these types of infectious diseases, were the hardest hit – along with the elderly and young children. The civilian population was also affected, with 25% of the population affected – New York lost 33,000 people and Philadelphia lost approximately 13,000.

HIV/AIDS

Human Immunodeficiency Virus (HIV) is an infection that attacks the body's immune system and Acquired Immunodeficiency Syndrome (AIDS) is the most advanced stage of the disease. HIV attacks the body's white cells (WBC), weakening the immune system – causing the individual to become sick with infection, tuberculosis, and some cancers. It is spread from the body fluids of an infected individual – i.e., from blood, breast milk, semen, and vaginal fluids. It is not spread by kisses, hugs, or sharing food. HIV can be treated and prevented with anti-retroviral treatment (ART). Untreated HIV can progress to AIDS, often after many years.

The global epidemic of HIV/AIDS is an ongoing worldwide health issue. The World Health Organisation (WHO) figures for 2022 indicate that the number of deaths is 40.4 million so far with ongoing transmissions in all countries globally. Some countries (particularly in Africa) are reporting increased trends in new infections when previously, they were on the decline. At the end of 2022, an estimated 39 million people were living with HIV, two-thirds of whom (25.6 million) were in the WHO African Register.

There is no cure for HIV infection. However, with access to effective HIV prevention, diagnosis, treatment, and care, HIV has become a manageable chronic health condition, enabling people living with HIV to lead long and healthy lives. By 2025, 95% of all people living with HIV (PLHIV) should have a diagnosis – and 95% of those should be taking lifesaving anti-retroviral treatment (ART), and 95% of PLHIV on treatment should achieve a suppressed viral load for the benefit of the person's health and for reducing untoward HIV infection.

When considering all people with HIV some 86% knew their status, 76% were receiving anti-retroviral treatment, and 71% had suppressed viral loads.

CHAPTER 6
EFFECTS OF WAR

War can have a dramatic effect on populations – and as we know can lead to tragic deaths and horrendous casualties. The younger generation will know about the Israeli-Hamas War in Gaza, the Ukraine War, and maybe the War in Afghanistan – but sadly few know about the wars of the last 200 years. Only the other month I had a visit by a younger generation couple – the chap's father used to visit my neighbour when he owned my house. The family was well connected in Germany, having owned a Schloss in a major town on the Rhine, and this youngster was university-educated. He was naturally interested in this house which his father regularly visited. I took him around and he was very interested in a black and white photo showing Field Marshall Viscount Montgomery in one of the dressing rooms. It was a photograph of which I am very proud, showing "Monty" and I with him signing a book, "Path to Leadership" on the bonnet of his car (Rolls Phantom c1936). The German youngster (aged 30) asked who that was. I was surprised he did not recognise him, so aptly I asked about Rommel, the German commander in North Africa in World War II, and he said he had never heard of him. I found this incredible and it is amazing how comparatively recent famous people are forgotten. For the younger generation, we were beaten back across the whole of North Africa by Rommel's Afrika Corps, until Montgomery's stand at El Alamein. Montgomery saved the day with excellent strategy and, as I learned only a few years ago, the supply for more tanks landing at Alexandria. Had we lost at El Alamein the Germans would have advanced on Iraq and seized our oil supply ... and in all probability, we would have lost the War.

It is worth looking at the wars of the last 200 years, looking first at World War I (WWI) and World War II (WWII) deaths – then the US involvement in wars and other significant wars.

WWI and WWII DEATHS

WWI   886,000
            (12.5% of those serving)
            (Also 6% of the adult population)
WWII   384,000 deaths
            (70,000 civilians)

You will note the deaths were much greater in WWI and this included trench warfare and shelling – many of the soldiers were effectively "cannon fodder". The confirmed casualties of WWII were 70,000 with 40,000 occurring in the nine months of the Blitz between September 1940 and May 1941.

In WWI the British population was 46.1 million, mobilised 6.1 million soldiers and 750,000 died. France had a population of 39 million, mobilised 8.1 million, and 1.34 million died.

WARS IN THE LAST 200 YEARS
In the last 200 years, the most important wars have been:

Napoleonic Wars	1 million–1.25 million deaths
Crimean War	2,500 British deaths
China Opium Wars	Virtually no deaths
China Civil War (Taiping Rebellion) (1850–64)	20 million–30 million
US Civil War	620,000
Anglo-Boer War	22,000 British soldiers died
World War I	886,000
World War II	384,000
Korean War	1,100 British deaths
Falklands War	255 British deaths
Iraq War	179 British deaths
Afghanistan War	405 British deaths

NAPOLEONIC WARS
I was taught about this in school but at no time did I realise the enormous numbers of deaths – greater than WWI and WWII combined. The figures are difficult to establish but nowadays, it is thought the Imperial Wars over 10 years cost 1 million–2.5 million lives. In Napoleon's Russian Campaign, some 30,000–50,000 soldiers deserted. Certainly, France, Britain, Russia, Prussia, Austria, and Spain each lost more than 100,000 – some many times more. In the Battle of Waterloo (1815), the amount of

French killed and wounded (captured) was 25,000. The British lost 3,500 and the Prussian army lost 1,200.

Throughout the campaigns, significant deaths were due to infection, related to living in close quarters and poor insanitary conditions. Also, wound infection carried a high mortality.

CRIMEAN WAR

The Crimean War (1853–56) was fought between Russia and an alliance of the Ottoman Empire (Turkey), Great Britain (UK), France, and Sardinia. The British lost 2,500, the French 1,700, and the Russians 12,000. One spin-off from the war was Florence Nightingale's work at the British base of Scutari, to which Crimean soldiers were sent, and this, of course, led to modern-day nursing practice. I have seen the building from a boat in the Black Sea. Part of Nightingale's ethos was good hygiene and good ventilation of the wards which reduced cross-infection. With the recent history of the Ukraine War, one might say history repeats itself!

CHINA OPIUM WARS

When I was in school these were barely touched upon but I thought they were worth mentioning. There were two Opium Wars, which were trade wars and virtually no loss of life. The first Opium War (1839–42) was between the British and China. The Second Opium War (1856–60) involved the British and French against the Qing Imperial China. For justification of these wars the Europeans considered free trade and the protection of missionaries – but in truth these wars were to flood China with opium. I must stress there was little or no loss of life – so perhaps should not be in this book. However, in doing my research, I came across the Chinese Civil War (Taiping Rebellion) which I had never even heard of, and is very important. I would add that there is no tie-up between the China Opium Wars and the China Civil War, which I will now describe.

CHINESE CIVIL WAR (TAIPING REBELLION)

The Taiping Rebellion (1850–64) was one of the bloodiest wars in human history, the bloodiest Civil War, and the largest conflict of the 19th century. It was not discussed in my history lessons in school, which concentrated on English and European history. One was made aware of the American Civil War in passing but never any mention of this Chinese internal conflict.

This rebellion was a civil war between the Manchu-led Qing Dynasty and the Hakka-led Taiping. The war lasted from 1850 until 1864, when Tianjing fell.

The uprising was commanded by Hong Xiuqinon, an ethnic Hakka. He alleged being the brother of Jesus Christ. The goals of the Hakka group were religious, nationalistic, and political in nature. Hong sought the conversion of the Han people to the Taiping secret version of Christianity – to overthrow the Qing Dynasty, and thereby have a state transformation. The Taipings sought to change the moral and social order of China and establish the Heavenly Kingdom as an oppositional state based in Tianjing. They gained control of a significant part of southern China, and eventually had a population base of nearly 70 million people.

For over 10 years, Taiping armies occupied and fought across much of the mid and lower Yangtse valley. This turned into a civil war and involved most of central and southern China. It is regarded as one of the bloodiest wars in human history and 30 million people fled the conquered regions to other parts of China or foreign settlements. Both sides carried out great brutality. The Taiping soldiers carried out widespread massacres of Manchus, the ethnic minority of the ruling Imperial House of Aisin-Gloro. The Qing Government also engaged in massacres, most notably against the civilian population of the Taiping capital, Tianjing.

The Taipings were weakened by internal conflict and were defeated by decentralised provincial armies such as the Xiang Army commanded by Zeng Guofan. He moved down the Yangtze River, recaptured Anqing, and later besieged Nanjing in May 1862. He beheaded 8,000 soldiers who surrendered and 10,000 women were carried off as booty. After two more years, on 1st June 1864, Hong Xiuquan died and Nanjing fell within a month. The 14-year Civil War weakened the Dynasty but was an incentive for a period of successful reform.

AMERICAN CIVIL WAR

The American Civil War (1861–65) was associated with the loss of 620,000 soldiers – greater than their fatalities for World War I and II combined, but recall they did not enter WWI until 1917. Their loss in various wars is as follows:

American Revolution War (1775–83)	25,000
War of 1812 (against the British)	20,000
American Civil War	620,000
WWI 1917–18)	116,000
WWII (1939–45)	405,000
Korean War (1950–53)	36,000
Vietnam War (1954–75)	58,000
War on Terror (2001–2021) (Afghanistan. Iraq)	7,000

BOER WAR

The Boer War (1899–1902) involved the biggest deployment of British troops since the Crimean War and there were volunteers from the empire – Canada, Australia, and New Zealand. Winston Churchill (later Prime Minister in WWII) was involved in this war.

British and Empire troops amounted to approximately 500,000. Some 22,000 British soldiers died (recall Islawanda and Rorke's Drift), of which only 35% died in battle and 65% from disease. There were also 40,000 who were wounded. I must say that when I visited Islawanda it was one of two places in the world which I found atmospheric. One could imagine the Zulus coming in their masses through a gap in the hills on the right – and the British were overwhelmed by the numbers. We were due to see the film Zulu on the tour bus but unfortunately, the television was not working. I suggested we get it displayed in the hotel that evening but the courier said not possible. Nevertheless, I approached management and everybody enjoyed the film! At Rorke's Drift, there was a hill overlooking the station and a large force of Zulus overlooked the station but fortuitously, they spotted Chelmsford's relief column approaching. I saw the window in the station where a lot of hand-to-hand fighting occurred. After the battle, some 351 had been confirmed killed, and it is speculated that 500 more who were wounded were massacred.

In this war, some 6000–7,000 Boer soldiers were killed. Over 100,000 Boer civilians (mostly women and children) were forcibly relocated into concentration camps where 26,000 died of various causes. This was a stain on the British Empire – and not surprisingly led to great resentment by the Boer population. The great problem was they were basically small farmers living in scattered communities and knew the terrain incredibly well – I can understand the problem the British military faced.

KOREAN WAR

The Korean War (1950–53) has been described as the first "hot war" of the Cold War. North Korea invaded the South which precipitated the involvement of a United Nations-mandated multinational force. The UK participated in the conflict through the contribution to the UN force. Over 81,000 British service personnel were deployed – 1,100 were killed in action, there were 2,600 casualties and 1,060 suffered as prisoners of war. The Americans had sent a larger contingent and they lost 37,000 personnel.

FALKLANDS WAR

This occurred in April–June 1982 when the Argentinians invaded. During the war some 255 personnel died – Royal Navy 86, Army 124, Royal Marines 27, Merchant Navy 6, and Royal Fleet Auxiliary 4. Three Falkland islanders were killed. By comparison, 649 Argentinian military were killed.

It was interesting that we Brits sent P&O Canberra down to the Falklands, and I had only been on her the year before. When I subsequently visited the island, I came to realise that the Capital, Port Stanley, was just like a small English village and the Government house was like a small white detached middle-class house. I had the opportunity to visit various battle sites and after several years there were a lot of signs relating to land mine clearance.

IRAQ WAR

The Iraq War (2003–2009) led to 179 personnel deaths

AFGHANISTAN WAR

The Afghanistan War was 2009–2010 and was associated with the deaths of 405 personnel.

CHAPTER 7
THREE PHASES OF MEDICINE

Some authorities consider that medically, longevity should be divided into three phases. The first phase was the historic times when things were very basic. Then came the second and most important phase of medicine, from the 1800s to the present day.

SECOND PHASE OF MEDICINE

This is the period which saw Jenner's involvement in the research involving cowpox and smallpox and the development of the smallpox vaccine. The discovery of cholera being water-borne and bad sanitation causing the spread of the condition led to steps to eradicate the condition. In the Victorian era, there were two important developments – the development of the light microscope which led to the diagnosis of bacterial disease and the advances in nursing practice. This was largely due to Florence Nightingale's involvement in the Crimean War. Injured soldiers were moved to her hospital at Scutari. She encouraged fresh air in the wards with open windows, patient separation, and excellent hygiene. This reduced the infection risk and reduced cross-infection from one patient to another.

Before this major development of antibiotics, medics used various measures to protect against disease-causing bacteria. Strict hygiene was universally important and individual treatments were used for specific conditions. For example, tuberculosis – a bacterial infection of the lungs – could only be treated with fresh air and rest. If we go back in history, American readers will be interested to know that George Washington's brother contracted tuberculosis and was sent to Barbados to recuperate. Then George Washington went there and had an extensive stay – and whilst there he learned much about farming and estate management. I have visited the house and seen the bedrooms they used, the house being in The Garrison, Bridgetown. In the late 1800s and the first half of the 1900s, we in Britain had a number of tuberculosis sanatoria for isolation.

ANTIBIOTICS. The next major step was the development of antibiotics. Most people will not know about the first antibiotic – Salvarsan. This was produced in Germany in 1909 by the medical scientist Paul Ehrlich and was used to treat Syphilis. It was considered a wonder drug and he referred to it as "the magic bullet". At the time it became one of the most prescribed drugs in the world.

During the 1930s chemists in Germany, France, and Britain discovered a whole range of new and effective chemical antibiotics – these were called sulphonamides. May & Baker of Dagenham developed the sulphonamide M&B 593 which was first prescribed in 1938 to treat pneumonia. The most famous person to be treated with this drug was Winston Churchill who contracted pneumonia at the height of World War II.

PENICILLIN. The introduction of penicillin in the 1940s has been recognised as one of the greatest advances in therapeutic medicine. It is interesting to note that it was discovered by chance by Dr Alexander Fleming and it changed the course of medicine. In 1928 he returned from holiday and in his laboratory he found mould growing on a petri dish of staphylococcal bacteria. He noticed the mould seemed to be preventing the bacteria around it from growing. He soon identified the chemical that killed the bacteria and named it penicillin.

The next driving force was the Australian pathologist Howard Florey, who became Professor of Pathology at Oxford's Dunn School in 1935 – and later (1945) attained the Nobel Prize. Florey invited Ernst Chain, after fleeing Nazi Germany, to join his team in Oxford in 1936 – and later (1945) he shared the Nobel Prize. Florey needed to make penicillin and he recruited six women, nicknamed "Penicillin Girls" to farm the penicillin. Florey's first wife (Mary Ethel Florey) had followed him to Oxford from Australia. She supervised the clinical trials of penicillin conducted at the Radcliffe Infirmary, Oxford, at military hospitals, and at the Birmingham Accident Department.

The first person to receive penicillin was Albert Alexander, a 43-year-old policeman, who was treated with penicillin in February 1941. Apparently, he had scratched his face on a rose bush and the wound had become infected and the infection had spread. In the US, the first person to be successfully treated with US-made penicillin was Ann Miller. With extensive cooperation between the US and Britain, the US were able to play a major role in the production of the drug, thus making a life-saving substance in limited supply into a widely available medicine.

CURRENT SITUATION. Currently, we can treat most medical conditions, and surgery and anaesthetics have improved over the last 100 years. Infant mortality used to be a major problem increasing the death rate, and over the years great advances have been made in obstetrics so infant mortality is now very low.

Curtailment of infectious disease and the advance of vaccines have been very important, and we only have to look at the management of COVID-19 to see how complex medical issues can be and to realise debate can occur. This is not to say that I agree with the decisions taken by the government and Chief Medical Officer, and I personally support the comments made by learned signatories of the Great Barrington Declaration. The WHO did not agree, citing any scientific evidence, but perhaps all should look at Sweden, where there was no second lockdown and their results were better than ours – with far less trauma (including psychological through isolation) and with saving that country the equivalent of millions of pounds. There was agreement on this document by Donald Trump, some Conservative politicians and support given in the Wall Street Journal.

The Great Barrington Declaration was the current lockdown policy published in an open letter in October 2020 in response to the COVID-19 lockdown. It was signed by 1,120 medical and public health scientists, and the signatories included doctors from the University of Oxford, Stanford University, and Harvard University. It was drafted in Great Barrington, Massachusetts in the US. Such a learned document would have been available to the government and Chief Medical Officer. The document considered that current lockdown policies were producing devastating effects on short and long-term public health. They were well aware that vulnerability to death from COVID-19 is more than 1,000 times higher in the old and infirm than in the young. As immunity builds in the population, the risk of infection to all – including the vulnerable – falls. We know that the population will reach herd immunity – i.e., the point at which the rate of new infection is stable – and this can only be assisted by but is not dependent upon a vaccine. Our goal should be to minimise mortality and social harm until we reach herd immunity.

The document goes on to say the most compassionate approach that balances the risks and benefits of reaching herd immunity, is to allow those who are at minimal risk of death to live lives normally. This would enable them to build up immunity to the virus through natural infection, while better protecting those at highest risk. They regarded this as "Focused Protection".

To me, this document is very logical and was clearly backed by many top scientists in the field.

THIRD STAGE OF MEDICINE

We are at the dawn of a new era where we hope there will be genetic engineering to eliminate certain conditions.

A good example to consider is breast cancer. Some 55,000 women are diagnosed with this condition annually and there is currently a lot of research going on which could lead to new treatments. It is known that inherited mutations increase the risk of developing the disease. Tests can be done for a few known genetic faults but not for all the genetic faults. A fault in the BRCA1 gene raises the risk to 60–90% and a mutation in BRCA2 raises the risk to 45–85%. So if there is a family history of breast cancer in the mother, then there is a ring of logic to the daughter having a genetic investigation – particularly if the mother had breast cancer at an early age. The famous Hollywood star Angelina Jolie was told she had a BRCA1 mutation and wisely, she decided to have a double mastectomy

CHAPTER 8
MEDITERRANEAN DIET

The Mediterranean diet is used throughout the whole of the Mediterranean area and there are subtle variations from place to place. The diet includes lots of healthy foods like whole grains, fruits, vegetables, seafood, beans, and nuts. It is noticed that those on the diet are less likely to put on weight, probably because of less caloric intake. One could infer therefore that any overweight person should undoubtedly go on this diet. The diet is very healthy and should be followed, along with other features like having antioxidants, not adding sugar, and getting plenty of exercise and sleep. You should have intermittent fasting and the right food, provided by this diet. The American Heart Association recommends this diet for preventing coronary disease and stroke – remembering that coronary heart disease is the biggest cause of death in the world today.

EFFECT ON BLOOD SUGAR. Studies have shown that it may reduce fasting blood sugar levels, decrease insulin resistance (making insulin more effective), and reduce HbA1c, the blood test used to diagnose type 2 diabetes. So in simple terms, the Mediterranean diet might prevent diabetes.

PLANT FOODS WITH POLYPHENOLS. The Mediterranean diet is packed with fruit and vegetables. I recommend particularly plant foods with polyphenols – berries (blueberries, raspberries, and strawberries), red wine, olives and olive oil, beans, and vegetables such as chicory, red onion, and spinach. In this regard and following the research, this last summer I greatly increased my strawberry and raspberry intake – and for the last two years have been taking two tablespoons of olive oil, swilled down with orange juice, and having a regular red wine with the main meal of the day.

EATING "STRESSED" PLANTS. Eating plants that have been stressed in their lives are better and are rich in antioxidants/polyphenols. A lot of information about antioxidants is discussed in the chapter on red wine. The best red wines are thought to be when the plant has been starved of water and may even have fungus on it. Plants often do not have much stress – for example, if the plant is made to grow bigger and faster, perhaps with fertiliser, then for the farmer that product is more valuable to him and probably would have little antioxidant/polyphenol. If on the other hand, the plant is grown in a field organically, without pesticides, then those plants are more stressed. In terms of plants, whole fruit or vegetables, look for items that are organically grown and colourful, because those are more likely to contain polyphenols. It is not always easy to get these products.

OPTIONS WITHIN THE DIET. You may be wondering what foods I particularly like that are within the

Mediterranean diet, so I have decided to make a list of the most significant possible items. You may be well versed in the subject, in which case you can skip reading the options. For example, I may have two scrambled eggs on toast after my porridge for breakfast, and for a bit of variety I often have beetroot or tomatoes added – but I have decided some days to substitute this with fried mushroom and onion.

VEGETABLES – Tomatoes, broccoli, kale, spinach, onions, cauliflower, carrots, Brussels sprouts, cucumber, sweet potatoes, and turnips.

FRUITS – Apples, bananas, grapes, pears, strawberries, raspberries dates, figs, melons, and peaches.
NUTS AND SEEDS – Walnuts, almonds, macadamia nuts, hazelnuts, cashews, pumpkin seeds, and peanut butter.
LEGUMES – Beans, peas, lentils, pulses, peanuts, and chickpeas.
WHOLE GRAINS – Oats, brown rice, rye, barley, corn, buckwheat, wholewheat bread, and pulses.
FISH AND SEAFOOD – Salmon, sardines, trout, tuna, mackerel, shrimp, oysters, clam, crab, and mussels.
POULTRY – Chicken, duck, pheasant, and turkey.
DAIRY – Milk, cheese, and yoghurt
HERBS AND SPICES – Garlic, basil, mint, rosemary, and sage
HEALTHY FATS – Extra virgin olive oil (EVOO), olives, and avocados

CHAPTER 9

IMPORTANT FEATURES FOR LONGEVITY

I consider there are ten important things to improve longevity:
1. Not smoking and no vaping
2. Good diet and avoid obesity
3. Intermittent fasting – "timed eating"
4. Having anti-oxidants (red wine, dark chocolate, walnuts and peanuts, blueberries, raspberries, strawberries, etc.)
5. Good sleep
6. Exercise
7. Avoid stress
8. Positive social relationships
9. No binge drinking
10. Remain free of opioid addiction

Interestingly since writing the draft of my work, I read a paper presented (2023) to The American Society of Nutrition by Dr Xuan-Mai Nguyen from the University of Illinois, Urbana. He presented eight habits to follow – but there was no mention of intermittent fasting or antioxidants. I think these two are critically important but that said, the theme is the same. The findings were from a questionnaire of 720,000 US military veterans – with the group aged 40–99 tracked for up to eight years.

It was pointed out that all eight of their recommendations should be followed and the earlier in life you start the better – and interestingly if you made the change in your forties, fifties, or sixties it is still beneficial. Women with all eight of these habits at the age of 40 were shown to live to 88 years but with none of the good habits the life expectancy was 66 years. Men with all eight good habits at the age of 40 would be expected to live to 86 years and with none of the good habits the life expectancy would be 62 years.

In the study, there were 33,375 deaths so the details of those could be carefully analysed. Overall the results showed that keeping physically active, not smoking, and not being addicted to opioid drugs had the largest impact. Exercise reduced the risk of early death by 46%, not smoking by 29%, and avoiding opioid drugs by 38%.

AVOID SMOKING

Smoking reduces your life expectancy by 10 years and should be avoided. You will be biologically older than a person who has never smoked. You will look older and be older – shown by readout parameters in the laboratory and by using a DNA methylating clock.

Smoking is well-known to cause cancer of the lung but can also cause bronchitis and Chronic Obstructive Pulmonary Disease (COPD). Do you want to have difficulty doing daily activities? Eventually, you may become breathless and may gasp, and as the situation gets worse you may become breathless even walking to the bathroom. At night you may have to be propped up with pillows. Later, you may need home oxygen or even ambulatory oxygen.

Smoking is known to cause coronary heart disease (angina or heart attack) and can be associated with diabetes, and tuberculosis, and can even affect the immune system. Smoking has also been associated with rheumatoid arthritis.

So if you want to avoid disease, it is never too late to stop smoking! And vapes are not the answer.

VAPING

Some people think that vaping helps you quit smoking – but unfortunately, you may end up addicted to vaping instead. So vaping should be avoided and you should stick to the approved methods to stop smoking which include patches, inhalers, lozenges, and gum.

What is vaping? It is when you use a handheld electronic device to breathe a mist (vapour) into your lungs. An e-cigarette, vape pen, or other electronic nicotine delivery system heats a liquid which contains:
- Flavouring
- Nicotine – the additive and harmful substance which is in cigarettes.
- Propylene glycol and glycerin which are used to create a vapour.

E-liquids and flavourings have ingredients which include:
- Chemicals such as acetaldehyde and formaldehyde which can cause cancer.
- Chemicals known to cause lung disease such as acrolein, diacetyl and diethylene glycol.
- THC (Tetrahydrocannabinol) – the chemical in marijuana which causes a high
- Vitamin E acetate linked to lung injury
- Heavy metals like nickel, tin, lead, and cadmium
- Ultra-fine particles which can get deep into the lungs

Problems include:
- Asthma and possibly COPD
- Lung scarring. Diacetyl, a chemical used in some flavourings, can cause Bronchiolitis obliterans which causes narrowing of the bronchioles
- Nicotine is an e-liquid which can raise blood pressure and narrow arteries
- EVALI is e-cigarette or vaping-induced lung injury. It causes widespread damage to the lungs and gives symptoms like coughing, breathlessness, and chest pain.
- Nicotine is addictive – changing your brain so you want more and more.
- Some ingredients in e-liquid can cause cancer.

AVOID BINGE DRINKING

In my years of medical training, I came to realise that excessive alcohol can cause terrible damage, causing cirrhosis of the liver, heart disease, strokes, and some cancers.

Anecdotally about a year ago, my Norfolk pal informed me he often had a bottle of Moet champagne in the evening. I was amazed at this and he said, "My liver function test (LFT) is normal." In response, I said he must see his general practitioner and ask for a Gamma GT. I told him the basic LFT could well be normal but he needs a more sensitive test.

As he is very involved in the motor industry, with a sense of humour I said, "I am not talking about the Bentley Continental GT, but what you need is a Gamma GT test!" Within a few days, he came back to say it was sky-high (many hundreds). I said that if he carried on like that he would develop cirrhosis and would be dead in under 10 years! He followed my advice to stop and in 2–3 months the Gamma GT was normal. There is a serious lesson to learn from this.

In many countries alcohol is used socially and in many ways is an integral part of British society. It isn't uncommon for people to call in at a pub on the way home or go later in the evening to meet old friends. That is fine if the alcohol is taken in moderation. I have one to two glasses (usually one) of red wine per day with my main meal. If abroad in a hot climate, then I appreciate a cool beer.

Binge drinking is particularly bad. British men are the third biggest binge drinkers in the world with 46% having six or more alcoholic drinks on a single occasion. This is slightly behind Romania with 55% falling into this category, and Denmark with 49%. The international general average is 27%.

British women top the table for women binge drinkers in the world. One in four get drunk monthly thanks to a "ladette" culture. Some 26% admit to consuming six or more alcoholic drinks on a single occasion.

In 2021, Britons drank an average of 111 bottles of wine in a year. I usually get through one bottle of red each week. Those having 111 bottles per year are having just over two bottles a week and this is equivalent to 10 litres of pure alcohol. According to the OECD (Organisation for Cooperation), worldwide the average is 8.6 litres with Latvia top at 12.2 litres. Indonesia has the least, with 0.1 litres of pure ethanol equivalent.

Now for an anecdotal story. I had my Australian second cousin come to stay and basically, though retired, had had a responsible post arranging international air flights into Australia. I am saying this merely to show he was a responsible person. Before coming I asked what alcohol was the preference expecting to be told beer or lager, but was told white wine. I only have racks of red so I thought I had better buy in some white. On arrival, the chap said he would appreciate a glass of white which I duly provided. I then discussed why I took red wine (see later chapter on this) so he said he would love to try my special red. I duly opened and had a glass of red with my meal. To my surprise by the end of the evening, the white bottle was empty and most of the red. I was amazed at this and diplomatically asked how much he normally drinks. The reply was he only had alcohol three times a week … but if he takes that sort of amount then sadly he is a binge drinker, and there could be significant disadvantages.

CHAPTER 10
CURE OBESITY

From my youth there used to be an adage, "We are what we eat". To a certain extent it is true, but clearly, to prevent obesity there are many factors – good diet, good amount of exercise, movement, sleep well, etc. By good diet, I mean eating proper food and not junk food. The latter can be processed or ultra-processed food, which contains a lot of extra carbohydrates and extra calories. Ultra-processed food has little fibre and eating such food does not lead to food satisfaction (satiety).

Most people will not admit to being overweight, and sadly "obesity" is a term avoided and any discussion can lead to upset. Critical obesity is a very serious condition, particularly gross obesity, and the average member of the public does not realise this. It can cause mobility issues but very importantly, obesity is associated with reduced lifespan and the possibility of incurring many medical conditions including hypertension (uncontrolled blood pressure), coronary artery disease (angina and heart attacks), and stroke. Quite often obesity can be tied in with the development of diabetes, which is well-known to be associated with adverse health risks, particularly vascular problems (from feet and legs to the heart and brain).

EXCESSIVE CARBOHYDRATE

Excessive carbohydrate is often a major factor. When I was a medical registrar (speciality trainee ST in modern terminology) and a consultant physician, doing my clinic I would often come across a patient who was grossly overweight, perhaps referred because of hypertension (raised blood pressure), diabetes, or some problem related to narrow coronary arteries. I would always ask about occupations which could be anything from lorry driver to virtually any occupation, and if the patient was obese I would usually ask about diet. I would almost always hear the word "sandwiches", particularly at lunchtime. This is bread/carbohydrate intake which needs to be curtailed. I would always give dietary advice and interestingly, I never heard a patient discuss any fruit!

MEDICAL CONDITIONS

There are well-established medical conditions associated with obesity, including diabetes and myxoedema (hypothyroidism). The latter have an underactive thyroid and almost invariably are overweight, can be sluggish, constipated, etc. The TSH (thyroid stimulating hormone) level is raised, determined by a blood test and the T4 is low. When given L-thyroxine, the symptoms improve and the patient may start to lose weight. If the TSH is elevated and T4 is normal, they are "borderline" and need to be monitored by blood tests as they become truly hypothyroid in future.

DIETARY CONSIDERATION. Underestimating carbohydrate portions often happens, and it is so easy for this to occur. If you overeat 400–500 calories you will never lose weight. So the message is to watch the portions – particularly your bread and potato intake. I have reduced my bread intake to one or two slices per day and the potato is down to three medium-sized with a main meal.

With dieting there is metabolic repositioning. With a long-term calorie deficit for some time, the body auto-regulates, realises the reduced calorie intake and down-regulates the food needs. Effectively the body slows down the metabolism.

A study by Bouchard et al looked at "Identical twins – responses to eating in identical twins". They were given the same diet and training regime but those that moved more and stood up more had an overall higher calorie need and lost 18lb more in 90 days. So the message from this is to stay active throughout the day. This you will note is what a centenarian said, as reported in an earlier section. This means that if you are sedentary in an office for most of the day you ought to get up and walk for five minutes every half an hour. Perhaps you would use the stairs rather than the lift, and when shopping in a supermarket, park further away from the main entrance. Gardening is also good for you – and I certainly do plenty of that. It has been said that even fidgeting might help! So the basic take-home message is any movement is good as it is using up calories.

EXERCISE

Doing 30 minutes of walking a day is helpful.

Active cardio in the gym helps – and may include running or cycling. Many do not know that excess cardio can have negative consequences – by putting the body under too much stress causing the release of cortisol – which inhibits fat loss. Overall going to the gym is "an optional extra" – walking and general exercise are satisfactory. I do that and some gym activities with a pull-up bar and use some weights. I certainly recommend you have a pull-up bar and you could use a couple of weights anywhere in the house.

LACK OF PROTEIN

Many gymnasts want to be super-fit and have 10% body fat with good abs. But 93% of people attending the gym never lose weight. For years it has been known that bodybuilders increase their protein intake to increase muscle size. This is logical but I have only just come to terms with how protein boosts fat loss in many ways. It gives high satiety (food satisfaction) and is metabolically active, burning more calories compared to carbohydrates and fat. So now, I add 20g of protein powder to some orange juice once or twice per day, making an orange shake. A high protein diet increases fat loss (which I noted with the protein shakes) but interestingly, if associated with high dairy intake the effect on fat loss (including abdominal fat) is even greater. A low dairy intake can actually reduce muscle mass.

It is recommended to have 30–60g of protein per meal. With this regime, you can expect to lose significant abdominal fat – which would probably never be achieved without this knowledge.

PROTEIN FOODS

You should eat more protein foods such as eggs, meat, fish, and beans. Some are now advocating having white meat (chicken or turkey) rather than red meat – and with this in mind, I now have chicken about three or four times a week.

EGGS. In the 1960s, following the American Heart Association documentation, there was worry about eating eggs because of the cholesterol content and questions were raised whether they lead to coronary artery disease. This theory has now been discounted by research. A study in the medical journal Heart (2018) included half a million adults and it was found that people who ate eggs most days had a lower increase in heart disease and stroke than those who eat eggs less frequently.

It is considered safe to eat two or three eggs per day but it is reported most healthy adults can consume four eggs per day. However, some say that if you have raised cholesterol it would probably be advisable to limit to four or five eggs per week. I must point out that with two or three eggs per day, the LDL (bad cholesterol) is not affected and there is an increase in HDL (good cholesterol). I would also point out that they contain all nine essential amino acids as well as vitamin D which improves the immune system. They also improve satiety (food satisfaction).

PROTEIN-RICH BREAKFAST

This is certainly a good idea and the scientific reasoning for this is analysed in a paragraph to be read shortly. I have a bowl of porridge oats each morning, which is a good source of protein, with blueberries on top (a rich source of antioxidants) and accompanied by a handful of walnuts (more antioxidant). I usually follow this with two scrambled eggs on toast giving me a good protein input. Occasionally I like a slice of smoked salmon, giving yet more protein. Historically, I always had cornflakes (popular years ago for my generation) and sometimes I would have a full English with egg, bacon, and tomato. It is worth noting an egg gives 7g of protein and two rashers of bacon give 16g of protein. I consider my current regime much healthier. Having protein at breakfast reduces the possibility of hunger mid-morning.

LUNCH/EVENING MEAL

You might have lamb, beef, pork, chicken, or fish – but remember white meat and fish are the healthier options. As a youngster I only had fish occasionally, probably once a week, but in the last year or so I have cut out lamb chops (previously my favourite) and now my main meal is most frequently chicken or fish – having fish as main course four times a week. If you are vegetarian, remember beans and lentils are packed with protein. One cup of lentils (200g) gives 20g of protein.

SCIENTIFIC STUDY RELATING TO PROTEIN

Some years ago, two professors at the University of Sydney set up a study recruiting 22 healthy volunteers who were put up in hotel-style accommodation within the University. They were split into two groups and each group was given different amounts of protein.

When on the low protein diet the participants ate on average 210 calories more per day than those on the higher protein diet. It was interesting to note they felt much more hungry with the lower protein diet, almost certainly because they had less protein which is thought to produce satiety (food satisfaction). Research has shown that it is best to spread the protein across the day rather than eating it all at once.

OBESITY ASSOCIATED WITH BREAST CANCER AND UTERINE CANCER

Obesity in women – having a body mass (BMI) greater than 30 – increases the risk of cancer of the breast and cancer of the uterus (endometrial carcinoma), with obese people being a third more likely to develop cancer of the breast.

The mechanism behind this is that fat cells produce an enzyme which raises the level of the hormone oestrogen. This hormone makes the cells in the breast and in the uterus divide more rapidly increasing the possibility of developing a tumour.

After menopause, oestrogen levels naturally fall but if the woman is overweight then there is still an excess of hormone circulating in the body. Also, it is worth noting that after menopause, levels of the hormone progesterone – which protects against excess oestrogen – fall. So obese women in middle age are putting themselves at great risk – and it is worth noting that 95% of uterus cancer is diagnosed in women over the age of 50. For the record, the main symptom is heavy or irregular bleeding, particularly after menopause. However, 80% of patients with uterus cancer now live for a decade or more having had appropriate treatment – which nowadays is usually removing the uterus with keyhole surgery.

The take-home message given this scenario, is that middle-aged women who are obese need to take action. Some research interestingly reports that if a woman has precancerous changes in the womb lining, losing weight might reduce this. However, I use the term "**might**" and expert gynaecological specialist management is needed.

CHAPTER 11
INTERMITTENT FASTING

This is probably the most important chapter in this book. Intermittent fasting is sometimes referred to as "timed eating" and is a comparatively new concept. It is the best thing you can do for general health and longevity. The best regime is probably a 16:8 intermittent fasting schedule, when there is an "eight-hour window" in which to eat. I note that Professor David Sinclair, a top geneticist at Harvard personally uses this regime. The regime is not set in stone as some authorities think the fasting period should be longer, maybe two to three days. Sinclair apparently tried fasting for three days but he reported this made him aggressive. Interestingly he noted the same effect in mice after three days. Sinclair decided he would not try that again and has made comments such as two meals a day (within the eight-hour window) might be a good option.

    I believe Sinclair sometimes uses two meals a day, skipping breakfast, and then eating lunch and evening meals (keeping the eight-hour window). Knowing that fasting is a crucial mechanism, he has suggested you might adopt his latest concept and occasionally miss food for one day. I personally am keeping to the eight-hour interval for eating, and it is not always easy to keep to this. I have noticed that I am not particularly hungry at breakfast so a lunch and meal later may be the best way for me to go, as Sinclair is currently doing. If you are working or on shifts, you will need to think carefully about how to sensibly incorporate a regime – and I must say I think two meals a day rather than three is the probable solution. Hotels and cruise ships have not adapted to this … but maybe one will have to deviate from the regime suggested for those periods!

It is probably advisable to keep the carbohydrate intake down to 1,000 calories per day – i.e., avoid some carbohydrates. Some have suggested reducing the calorie intake by 75% for two days a week – but I think I might occasionally miss a day's food.

AUTOPHAGY

You probably have not heard of this scientific term. Autophagy is a process activated by intermittent fasting which promotes good health. This is the body's mechanism for recycling old or damaged cells and it has been linked to many health benefits such as increased lifespan and can protect against diseases such as cancer.

It is important to note it is not just what you eat but when you eat – and the latter probably has greater significance than the former, but both are critical. The period of not eating is the main factor to boost the body's defences against ageing to promote longevity. Stress from fasting triggers a metabolic shift in your genes, up-regulating sirtuins and AMP (see previous chapter on

Genetics) and down-regulating mTOR. Insulin sensitivity is also turned on. To me, the complex scientific evidence seems fairly clear-cut.

HISTORICAL CONCEPT

When we were cavemen and hunter-gatherers we lived in adversity. We had to do a lot of exercise, maybe hunting or running away from predators, and we could only eat when food was available.

The present-day lifestyle is not what the human body was designed for and is far too comfortable. Many do not get enough exercise, taking the car rather than walking, using the escalator rather than stairs, and sitting at the desk for hours. At the airport recently this went through my mind, virtually nobody choosing the stair option! We may have an office job and not move from the desk for hours. We may have three meals a day, and maybe an odd snack as well. This does nothing for our health and longevity, and we need:

- Walking and exercise
- Gym activity
- Intermittent fasting

RELIGIOUS GROUPS

Interestingly over the centuries, some religious groups have practised fasting. Ramadan – the ninth month in the Islamic calendar – is one of the most sacred for Muslims. During the month they are not allowed to eat or drink, not even water, during daylight hours. In other words, once a year for one month, they are effectively doing a 16-hour fast per day. So with my regime of a 16-hour fast every day, I am doing this overnight – but Muslims are doing this in the daytime but for only one month a year.

WESTERN CULTURES

For a long time, these have followed a three-times-a-day regime. This was instilled into me as a child, being told to have a good breakfast and not to skip meals. Only recently I read but had not realised, that the Pilgrim fathers took the three-times-a-day regime to America when they landed in Plymouth, Massachusetts, in 1620. Before this, in the Middle Ages, the upper classes sometimes had severe gluttony – taking King Henry VIII as an example with his enormous meals and rotund features. Throughout the Victorian era (1837–1901), and the Edwardian Era (1902–10) subsequently three times a day meals were the norm – and it was usual to have a light lunch and large evening meals.

CALORIC OVERLOAD

It is now recognised that three main meals a day is a caloric overload, even in children. If a child is carrying excessive fat then the child is being overfed. These effects may have an effect on the child for years. The epigenetic memory of being obese as a child can affect the future lifestyle.

PHYSIOLOGY OF FASTING

Basic physiology is when we eat carbohydrates they are broken down into sugar – needed by the cells for energy. Any excess energy is stored in the fat cells and these sugars can only be released from the fat cells if the plasma insulin falls low enough. Every time we eat or snack there is an insulin spike – effectively stopping sugar from being released from the fat cells. With a stretch of fasting the insulin level stays lower for longer and the fat can be burnt off. This is a critically important mechanism.

When we are not eating overnight (i.e., fasting) the body has a rest or "clean-up" period, which is now referred to as autophagy.

In the NE Journal of Medicine (1019), it is noted that fasting for 18 hours and eating in "a six-hour window" changes the metabolism from glucose-led to ketone-based energy, This report indicates that this increases longevity, and stress resistance, and lowers the incidence of obesity and cancer.

CHAPTER 12
SOME FOODS TO AVOID

The main foods to avoid are:
- Sugar
- Margarine
- Processed meats – bacon and sausage
- Ultra-processed foods
- Some bakery products
- Modern wheat

SUGAR

My personal advice is you should stop taking sugar, even if you wean yourself off slowly over two or three months. As a teenager many years ago I always had two spoonfuls of sugar in tea and coffee and in my early 20s, there were reports that it was not good for you. I weaned myself off quickly in the case of tea but with coffee, I needed one tablespoonful for about six weeks, then half a tablespoonful and then stopped. If you are healthy, with normal body weight and no disease, you can probably eat 10–20g of sugar per day and remain healthy. Guidelines say 50g per day but some authorities think this is too much. Many eat

100g per day and this is causing degenerative disease and mental disease. The general advice should probably be to avoid adding sugar.

The genetic mechanism involving sugar is known by few people, mainly geneticists and scientists. At a high level glucose shuts off the body's protective mechanisms – AMPK and sirtuins (discussed in the Genetics chapter). If you eat three meals a day, your glucose will spike and your defences against ageing are going to be working at a minimum. You need to adjust your diet to avoid these spikes, and this can be achieved by intermittent fasting (an eight-hour window for eating and nothing for 16 hours).

Metabolism. Sugar is a natural molecule but it is empty calories – with no real nutritional purpose and does not give satisfaction (satiety). For many years I thought sugar was all glucose but the truth is that 50% of sugar is glucose and 50% is fructose. Consumption of glucose causes a rise in blood glucose, which causes an insulin spike which then causes a drop in the blood glucose. In simple terms, the "insulin system" gets worn out and so-called insulin resistance may occur and this can lead to pre-diabetes and diabetes mellitus.

Sugary cereals are very popular with children and we now know that sugary foods, with all the fibre stripped out, can cause inflammation. In my childhood, with a strict three-times-a-day meal regime, I always had Kellogg's cornflakes for breakfast. These were incredibly popular in that era. Out of interest I recently decided to look up the sugar content of my childhood staple and compare it with porridge oats. I was amazed to discover that Kellogg's cornflakes have 8g of sugar per 100g and porridge oats had less than 0.5g per 100g. Some years ago I thought it was sensible to change to muesli, but muesli with dried fruit has a lot of sugar. If you buy prepared muesli it may have up to 26g of sugar in one cup. Needless to say, about three years ago I changed over to regular porridge oats for breakfast because I realised this is an excellent food and contains a lot of fibre. It is almost certainly the top choice for breakfast – when it is made with low-fat milk or water. All porridge oats are whole grains and they contain a lot of soluble fibre called beta-glucan, which can help lower your cholesterol and the fibre helps the gut microbiome. This feeds the probiotics of the gut – and this keeps the immune system strong and healthy. Do not add sugar or salt, or you will undo all the good work. Some add a banana but a few years ago somebody on the internet was taking blueberries. I found this an excellent idea as they are full of antioxidants (discussed later in the book) and at the same time, I eat a handful of walnuts (again full of antioxidants). Overall I find I buy a packet of walnuts per week – a good investment!

FRUCTOSE

Many people will not realise that 50% of sugar is fructose, It is a greater problem in the US compared to the UK, as it is very common in the American diet with the introduction of cheap high fructose corn syrup (HFCS) in the 1970s to act as a substitute for cane sugar. In the US it is widely used to sweeten a variety of foods, including soda, candy, baked goods, and cereals. Excessive HFCS have been linked in studies to obesity, diabetes, and heart disease.

Fructose does not raise blood sugar (as blood sugar here equates to blood glucose) but causes the metabolic condition of Non-Alcohol Fatty Liver Disease (NAFLD). This can be associated with obesity and the disease can cause liver inflammation and liver damage, which result in a more aggressive disease called non-alcohol steatohepatitis (NASH). This can progress to liver scarring (cirrhosis), liver cancer, and liver failure.

High levels of fat in the liver are associated with hypertension, heart problems, diabetes, and kidney disease. Professor Sanyal published a paper in the New England Journal of Medicine in which he did a four-year follow-up of cases with biopsy-proven NAFLD and he found the most common problem was new onset hypertension followed by type 2 diabetes, chronic kidney disease (CKD), extra-hepatic cancer, and liver cirrhosis.

Fructose causes obesity. Scientists from the University Anschutz School of Medicine (US) published a paper on obesity. They investigated how fructose affects cells and they considered fructose, unlike other cells, causes our metabolism to go into "a low power mode". This causes hunger and so we eat more (not just sugary foods), despite having eaten plenty. The normal physiology of the gut is that when we eat food it is broken down in the gut and then converted to ATP (adenosine triphosphate), which every cell in the body uses as its energy source. In this obesity paper, the authors claim that if you eat too much fructose, this suppresses the production of ATP. With the falling ATP levels, the body thinks the energy supply is at risk and this triggers hunger signals which encourage you to eat more – hence this could be the mechanism for obesity.

There is also a very interesting paper relating to obesity coming from the NY-Presbyterian/Cornell Medical Centre which published a paper in 2019. The researchers divided mice into three groups – the first group was put on a low-fat diet, the second group on a high-fat diet, and the third on a high-fat diet with added fructose. Those mice with added fructose to the diet put on a lot of weight compared to the other two groups. Interestingly and importantly in that group, they found that the villi of the small intestine – finger-like projections that line the wall of the bowel and are responsible for absorption – were much longer. It was therefore postulated that this is the mechanism that shows why this group absorbed more calories, with consequent obesity. Interestingly the same team has also shown that feeding fructose to mice encourages cell growth, and they thought this might be the cause of occasional colorectal cancer.

So the take-home message is to avoid fructose and all sugar!

MARGARINE

In my youth, a lot of people changed over from butter to margarine because it was thought to be more healthy. My family kept to traditional butter. With current evidence, my personal view is that margarine should avoided at all costs

In manufacture, there is partial hydrogenation (i.e. bombarded with hydrogen) and in doing so trans-fats are created, which are unsaturated but behave like saturated fat. With these different fats, the difference is with the biochemistry:

Fatty acids – long chain of carbon
with hydrogen on each side

Trans-fats have a carbon double bond
instead of a single carbon.

The next bit is a bit complicated but is critical to understand. Basically, nature makes trans-fats differently from those that are manufactured. Apparently in nature, the carbon double bond is at the 11th position in the chain but man-made trans-fats have the double bond in the 9th position. This makes all the difference. Man has had the right enzymes for natural trans-fats for thousands of years but we do not have the ability to deal with the new man-made trans-fats.

Manufacturers claim their trans-fats are cheap and promote the shelf-life, and indeed can be on the shelf for a long time. They comment the product has a good texture and overall saves money. Some companies use the term "trans-fat free per serving" but in fact have less than 0.5g – i.e. the trans-fat per portion which is considered acceptable. But, despite these comments, we should go back to the basic biochemistry discussed, noting we do not have the enzymes to deal with these new products!

The bad fats affect the blood vessels, creating the possibility of narrowing the coronary arteries and this increases the blood glucose levels. This causes diseases including metabolic syndrome obesity, hypertension, and diabetes in the same patient.

UNHEALTHY PROCESSED FOODS

Processed foods generally have been altered in preparation, whether by freezing, canning, baking, or drying. Some processed foods contain high levels of fat, salt, and sugar. Some processed foods are good for us – for example, frozen vegetables and frozen fruit – often frozen at the time of freshness. Canned produce can be a good, affordable way to get your vegetables but if you can, choose fresh or frozen. Unhealthy processed foods should be avoided, the main ones being:

- Sweetened coffee and tea
- Energy drinks and soft drinks
- Sausages, hot dogs and deli meat
- Frozen pizza and frozen meals
- Packaged snacks such as crisps, crackers and cookies
- Most breakfast cereals
- Canned or instant soups
- Sweetened yoghurt

BAKERY PRODUCTS

Bakery products such as doughnuts, brownies, and cookies are not a good idea. They contain excess sugar and no fibre. Consumption of sugar spikes glucose and insulin levels – and the excess sugar gets converted into fat and can cause obesity. Visceral fat around the middle occurs and internally there can be increased fat around various organs. The excess sugar causes an increase in LDL-C (bad cholesterol) and increased triglycerides – both adverse factors for coronary artery disease. So if you are going to eat bakery products go for whole-grain pastries, with nuts and seeds.

MODERN WHEAT

Modern wheat can be a problem but is difficult to avoid. Overall one might say that modern wheat has helped society generally and tens of thousands of types of wheat have been developed by scientists. With these modern wheats, scientists have looked at:
- resistance to weather
- resistance to drought
- resistance to strong winds
- what is the yield per acre

These seem to be the driving forces and the scientists are not involved in how humans will tolerate them. So one does not know precisely what bread one is buying but I would advise you to buy home-baked bread or seeded farmhouse loaves where possible.

It is worth documenting Coeliac Disease which is an intestinal condition due to an allergy to gluten (found in wheat). The inflammatory process affects the epithelial lining of the intestinal wall, causing the cells to become stubby and flattened rather than tall and elongated. Associated with this, the patient gets loose stools and abdominal distension. The diagnosis is usually confirmed histologically and a gluten-free diet works wonders for controlling the disease.

CHAPTER 13
ANTIOXIDANTS

I want to discuss the following in relation to antioxidants:
- Red wine
- Grapes
- Blueberries
- Raspberries and strawberries
- Walnuts
- Dark chocolate
- Olive oil
- Tea
- Red cabbage
- Beetroot
- Spinach and kale

RED WINE

About seven years ago, I read an interesting Sunday Times article about a village in France in the Pyrenees, very close to the Spanish border, where men drink the local wine and live for 105–115 years and have no coronary artery disease, no strokes, and no dementia. In fact, they have the greatest longevity in the whole of Europe. As a consultant physician, I was intrigued and wondered why this was the case. I thought I must investigate further and this led me to consider the overall package for longevity. Part of this study was out of self-interest and preservation, but I wanted to get to the bottom of the whole saga. After very extensive investigation I thought I should impart the knowledge to help others who are interested in living longer and healthily.

I think the critical feature is the presence of antioxidants, particularly Resveratrol – and in my view, this increases longevity. About the time of reading about this village and its wine, I attended a medical conference on a Saturday morning and remember sitting in the front and an eminent Professor from Birmingham made the statement, "The answer to longevity is nuts." The Press got hold of that on the Monday! Well, it is partly true that walnuts have a high concentration of ant-oxidant, so there is a common theme with the wine. If the ladies, on the other hand, want shiny hair – go for Brazil nuts!

Sirtuins. Years ago (about the year 2000) it was discovered that the enzyme sirtuin controls ageing. Activation of this enzyme (paper by Loe) slows ageing. It was discovered that polyphenol molecules in plants activate sirtuin (Loe & Howard paper, Harvard University) with a 10% increase in activity. The main polyphenol is Resveratrol (2003 Sinclair paper, Harvard) and binding to the sirtuin renders the latter hyperactive. As an anecdote it is worth noting that Resveratrol given to mice daily gives the best life extension even if they have a fat diet. Subsequently, these findings have been substantiated. It is now accepted that sirtuins protect the body against toxins, inflammation, and damage. It is interesting to note that in the laboratory, mice that were given a high-fat diet plus Resveratrol were as healthy as mice on a healthy, lean diet.

HORMESIS IN PLANTS. This is a term which you may not have heard of. Hormesis is important when you put the body under stress, making it perceive it might not survive, and this happens with severe exercise and intermittent fasting. In the same way, it applies to plants and some authorities think we should eat plants that have been stressed. These tend to be full of colour. As an anecdote, you would not pick grapes after a bout of rain. The plant needs to be "stressed" as if it might die, and it then produces the antioxidant chemical Resveratrol, which is in the skin of the grape. The skin of the grape is left in the fermentation process for red wine, but most people do not know that in the manufacture of white wine, the skin is removed (hence the white colour). So white wine has a different chemical composition from red wine. My personal take on this is that the critical antioxidant is in red wine and white wine has nothing like the advantage of red wine. I remember in my late teens and early 20s when I drank wine, I chose a sweeter white, but after stopping sugar I no longer liked the taste so moved on to a dry white. Now more recently, for the last seven years or so, since the Sunday Times article, I only drink red wine – mainly from the village in the Pyrenees.

Village in the Pyrenees. So I have already stated the greatest longevity in Europe is in a little village in the Pyrenees near the Spanish border. I gather the elderly gentlemen meet each day for lunch – so having good social contact. They have a Mediterranean diet, which in itself is good, but also one or two glasses of red wine and French cheese. You might say the cheese is not so healthy, but remember the experiment on mice where the high-fat negative effect was nullified by Resveratrol. The men live to 105–115 years and have no coronary artery disease, no strokes, and no dementia. They are also remarkably fit. The pundits might say they have the Mediterranean diet but so does the whole of the Mediterranean littoral. I think the mechanism for their success is the red wine.

Now, why is this village so special? It is because they ferment the grapes for 11 months, not the usual six and the process leads to a high Resveratrol (a polyphenol) content. I was amazed when I read about this duration of fermentation. In fact, the wine has been chemically analysed and it has been shown to have the highest possible concentration of antioxidants.

It is interesting to note that in Europe, the second-longest longevity is in a village in Sardinia – although Sardinia overall has good longevity. The common denominator is that this particular village ferments the grape for 11 months, as in the French village. This seems to be more than just a coincidence.

I well remember years ago being on a small boat going up the coast of Croatia and over the tannoy the lady started to praise the local wine and said how they ferment it for six months. I thought that was nothing unusual, as that is the practice across the globe. It made me cast my mind back to the then-recent French Pyrenees story.

Now for a very interesting and relevant anecdotal story. About three years ago, I was helping to run an acute medical assessment ward and was presented with a very slim, upright 102-year-old who seemed very sprightly. The junior staff had clerked her in – "clerking" being an old term for writing the case up with history, examination and diagnostic conclusion. Recently of course this is now often done on the computer on wheels. In the social history, the junior doctor asked about smoking and she said she had given that up at 62 because she realised it was not healthy. They had correctly asked about alcohol and she said she would drink one to two glasses per day. The juniors gave me this history and I walked along to see her, introduced myself and said my staff had told me a lot about her.

I did not say the information given but asked an open-ended question, "What do you attribute your longevity to?" She then gave me the smoking and alcohol story. Normally with that information, no further question would be asked in that regard but with my recent interest in longevity, I asked her what wine she drank.

She replied proudly, "Oh, I drink my husband's wine." Not many doctors would ask my next question which was how long did he ferment it for. To my surprise, she said, "For 18 months." In other words, he was effectively feeding her antioxidants. I think I have never seen such a sprightly centenarian. She had pneumonia, which we treated, and she was transferred from the admission unit to a general medical ward – and I do not know the outcome.

It often takes a lot to convince me of a new hypothesis but I am sold on the antioxidant effect, and benefit of certain red wines. I drink one or two glasses of red wine from the specific village in the Pyrenees and I hope this keeps me fit and healthy.

Other antioxidants. Grapes are rich in many

antioxidants including Resveratrol, Catechins, epicatechins, and Proanthocyanidins. It is thought they all give health benefits and have a protective effect against developing type 2 diabetes. This is because red wine contains Resveratrol and curcumin, which have anti-inflammatory and anti-diabetic properties. A study in the journal "Agriculture and Food Chemistry" found that polyphenols in red wine inhibit the activity of alpha-glucosidase, an enzyme that breaks down carbohydrates into glucose.

Carbohydrate ------||-------- glucose
Alpha-glucosidase
Blocked by polyphenols

The study involved 200 type 2 diabetic patients. They were split into three groups:
1. one glass of red wine per day
2. one glass of white wine per day
3. given water

All had a healthy Mediterranean diet without calorie restriction. At two years, it was noted that the red wine group had lower overall cholesterol and increased HDL cholesterol (good cholesterol) and there was better blood sugar control. The conclusion reached was that drinking small amounts of red wine reduced heart disease risk and, apart from the good effect on HDL, there was better next morning fasting blood sugar.

GRAPES

Grapes are a popular fruit that is rich in antioxidants – and we have already discussed this in the section on red wine. New research in the Scientific Journal of Food and Nutrition (Jung Kim) found that elderly people who ate a cup and a half of grapes regularly could improve eye health with better vision. It is the first study of its kind and it was found that older people who ate a cup and a half of grapes daily over four months improved their eye health. The researchers looked at improvement in macular pigment accumulation – noting macular pigment optical density (MPOD).

BLUEBERRIES

Blueberries have the highest amount of antioxidants among fruits and vegetables. They contain anthocyanins which are said to reduce the risk of heart disease.

RASPBERRIES AND STRAWBERRIES

Raspberries are described by some as a superfood as they contain a large number of antioxidants and vitamin C. Half a cupful has 25% of the recommended vitamin C intake per day and this slows down the ageing process with fewer skin wrinkles and protects the immune system. They also contain powerful anthocyanins which reduce oxidative stress and therefore lower the incidence of heart disease. There is an interesting study from 2010 which investigated a test tube containing numerous cancer cells. Some 95% of breast, stomach, and colon cancer cells were killed by the antioxidants from raspberries.

Strawberries are a very popular fruit and contain a lot of antioxidants and a very high concentration of vitamin C. The anthocyanins lower the level of "nasty" low-density lipoprotein (LDL cholesterol) and replace it with "good" HDL.

WALNUTS

Walnuts have the highest concentration of antioxidants in any nut. In fact, it is double that in any other nut. The polyphenols act against free radicals and reduce the risk of heart disease and various cancers. They should be eaten raw and uncooked as heating reduces the effects of the antioxidants.

DARK CHOCOLATE

Dark chocolate is very good for you as it contains a lot of antioxidants, dilates blood vessels, lowers blood pressure, and even decreases insulin resistance (possibly preventing type 2 diabetes) and is nutritious.

In my youth, I could not understand why people would buy expensive dark chocolate as opposed to ordinary chocolate bars. At that time we did not know about antioxidants. You really need to buy dark chocolate with 70% or 85% cocoa. I try to get the latter from a supermarket and I tend to buy the packet with five pieces (5 x 25g) in it and I have one packet a week. As an anecdote, it is reported that Queen Elizabeth the Queen Mother, who lived to 102, always had dark chocolate each night so she was giving herself antioxidants.

Antioxidant. Dark chocolate is rich in antioxidants including polyphenols, flavanols and catechins. Research has shown that polyphenols may lower LDL cholesterol (bad cholesterol) when combined with cocoa. One study interestingly showed that dark chocolate had even more antioxidant effects than blueberries (which are known to be high in antioxidants). In fact, dark chocolate may have more antioxidants than other foods.

When nasty LDL cholesterol oxidises, the particle becomes reactive and damages the inner lining (endothelium) of blood vessels. So by lowering the LDL, dark chocolate prevents damage to heart blood vessels – and therefore, has a preventative action against you developing angina or having a heart attack.

Dark chocolate lowers blood pressure by causing dilatation of blood vessels so it is good for cardiovascular health (both heart and peripheral blood vessels). One review study has shown that eating dark chocolate three times a week lowers the risk of cardiovascular disease by 9%. Another study suggested that eating 45g lowers cardiovascular risk by 11% but eating more than 100g per week does not lead to health benefits. This would only be four slices of my chocolate per week … so my five slices per week have me covered!

It also diminishes insulin resistance because it contains flavanol …. and this may stop you from developing type 2 diabetes.

Dark chocolate is very nutritious because it contains a lot of fibre and is rich in minerals – iron, magnesium, copper, and manganese – as well as potassium, phosphorus, zinc, and selenium. It also contains fats, mainly oleic acid (found in olive oil) and this is healthy. Dark chocolate also contains caffeine and theobromine, with caffeine acting as a stimulant. However, the amount is small compared to coffee, so does not affect your sleep pattern.

OLIVE OIL

Olive oil is a staple of the Mediterranean diet and is used throughout the whole Mediterranean littoral – with countries including France, Spain, Italy, Greece, Egypt, Tunisia, and Algeria. The people in the Mediterranean littoral who use olive oil have a higher life expectancy and lower risk of heart disease, hypertension, and stroke compared with the rest of the world.

Process. Olive oil is derived from the olive Olea Europaea and the process involves crushing ("cold pressing") whole olives into a paste without the use of heat or chemicals. The paste contains at least 30 beneficial plant compounds, many of which are antioxidants. Force is then applied to the paste by mechanical press or centrifugation to separate the oil from the pulp. Cold pressing enables the oil to retain its nutritional value – and the EU has set standards that the temperature must not exceed 21°C. Under higher heat, the nutrients and beneficial plant compounds can break down.

There are grades of olive oil, determined by the amount of oleic acid present. The highest grades are Extra Virgin and Virgin Oil. Experts agree that olive oil and in particular Extra Virgin Olive Oil (EVOO) is good for you. Extra Virgin Oil is the first pressed oil and no chemicals are added during the pressing.

Cooking. When olive oil or any cooking oil is heated to a point where it smokes, it breaks down and may produce potentially carcinogenic toxins – the smoke point of olive oil is about 200°C. Olive oil stands up well to heat and fares much better than other vegetable oils. At one stage it was debated that it was not a good idea to cook with Extra Virgin Oil but several studies over the years have proven this is simply untrue. Not only is EVOO safe to cook with but it is the most stable and safest cooking oil available.

Composition. Olive oil is nearly all fat – 73% of the fat is oleic acid, 11% polyunsaturated, and 14% saturated. Unsaturated fats are very advantageous – they are Omega 3 and Omega 3 fatty acids. Saturated fats are not good fats and olive oil contains 2g of saturated fat per 15ml. This is well within the recommended limit by most authorities. One critical fact is that olive oil contains antioxidants. You keep hearing about these in this book and I think there is a "theme" of connecting evidence of their benefit for longevity. The antioxidants help prevent heart disease (the main killer), diabetes, and cancer. Just 15ml of olive oil contains the recommended allowance of vitamin E – a potent antioxidant. It is also rich in the plant compounds oleuropein and hydroxytyrosol which are powerful antioxidants in animal and laboratory studies. This is probably the mechanism for the benefit of the Mediterranean diet.

Consumption. Extra Virgin Olive Oil (EVOO) may be used in cooking but a lot of Mediterranean people put it on salads, etc. If drinking olive oil it should be taken on an empty stomach, in the morning or before sleeping. I personally take two tablespoonfuls of olive oil neat before breakfast – but take it with half a glass of pure orange juice to prevent throat irritation.

Mechanism of action and benefits. The crucial factor, known by geneticists and some scientists, is that olive oil activates sirtuins (see chapter on Genetics). The consequential benefits are:
- Protects against heart disease
- May help prevent strokes
- Helps with diabetes and Metabolic Syndrome
- Helps with obesity
- Can help Rheumatoid Arthritis
- Effect on mental health
- Possible anti-bacterial property
- May help with cancer prevention
- May help with depression

Heart Disease. It protects against heart disease by preventing the oxidation of "nasty" LDL cholesterol, reduces inflammation (a driver in heart disease) and is said to lower blood pressure which is advantageous. It improves the lining of blood vessels. The Mediterranean diet, which relies on olive oil as its main source of fat, has been shown to reduce the incidence of heart attack and stroke by up to 28%.

May help prevent a stroke. Strokes can be due to a blood clot (cerebral thrombosis) or haemorrhage (bleeding). Olive oil helps prevent blood clots and helps the lining of blood vessels (i.e. in the brain and heart). The relationship between olive oil and strokes has been extensively studied. A large review of 841,000 people showed that olive oil was the only source of mono-unsaturated fat ("good fat") and this was associated with reduced risk of stroke and heart disease.

Helps with diabetes and Metabolic Syndrome. Olive oil has strong anti-inflammatory properties – and we know chronic inflammation is a driver of diseases such as cancer, heart disease, type 2 diabetes and Metabolic Syndrome ("trilogy" of obesity/diabetes/hypertension). Several studies have shown the beneficial effect of olive oil on blood sugar and insulin sensitivity – so this is a very important mechanism. One study found that a diet rich in olive oil reduces the risk of diabetes by 40%.

May help with obesity. I do not have any scientific papers on this but one should note there is less obesity among Mediterranean countries which consume olive oil.

May help in Rheumatoid Arthritis (RA) and Osteoarthritis (OA). Rheumatoid arthritis is an auto-immune condition with painful joints. Olive oil appears to reduce inflammatory activity, evidenced by the reduction of inflammatory markers ESR and CRP which clinicians use as indicators of inflammation. Some think that olive oil may delay the progression of OA. Animal studies have suggested that olive oil might fight OA by preventing cartilage damage, thus protecting joints.

Helps Mental Health. The MIND diet, which recommends cooking with olive oil, combines the Mediterranean diet with the Dietary Approaches to Stop Hypertension (DASH) diet. The MIND diet is high in vegetables, berries, nuts, whole grains, and fish. The MIND diet showed a slower decline in mental sharpness and memory with age. A study over four and a half years of 923 people found that this diet led to a 53% reduction in the rate of Alzheimer's.

Anti-bacterial activity has been suggested, postulating

that olive oil contains many nutrients that can inhibit harmful bacteria. One study suggested that 30g of olive oil can eliminate Helicobacter pylori (which can cause stomach ulcers) in two weeks. This however is not the conventional medical treatment but is an interesting finding and needs further studies.

May help prevent cancer. Some studies have suggested that olive oil can prevent numerous types of cancer – including breast cancer, bowel cancer, colon cancer, and child leukaemia. The cancer is caused by cell mutation and that can be related to toxins. To combat these toxins the body needs antioxidants and vitamins, like those contained in olive oil. The effect could be related to the mono-unsaturated fatty acids in olive oil that have been proven to lower the production of prostaglandins derived from arachidonic acid which plays a significant part in the production and development of cancerous tissue.

$$\text{Arachidonic Acid} \xrightarrow{\text{Olive Oil}} \text{Prostaglandins}$$
(Can produce tumours)

TEA

Tea is certainly very popular in the UK and is consumed by two-thirds of the world's population. We keep hearing about antioxidants (in red wine, berries, nuts, etc.) in this book and it is noted that tea contains antioxidants, and may reduce the risk of heart attacks and strokes. Much research has been done, particularly on green tea, which has health benefits with alleged cancer-protective properties.

A paper By Raederstorff DG et al in Nutrition Biochem 2003:14:326-32 noted that green tea catechins affected lipid metabolism in rats and prevented the appearance of atherosclerotic plaques. It is postulated that it decreases the absorption of triglyceride and cholesterol, but also increases the excretion of fat.

I have said that tea contains antioxidants and this seems to be the mechanism for the reduction of heart disease and vascular disease (including strokes). One study actually showed a nearly 20% reduction in heart attacks and a 35% reduced risk of strokes in those who drink three cups of green tea per day. Those who drank four cups or more had a 35% reduction in the risk of heart attack and lower levels of 'nasty" LDL cholesterol. Japanese researchers have found that green tea can decrease tooth loss because it changes the PH of the mouth (reducing acidity) and this may prevent cavities. This is interesting but one must never rely on just one study.

There are several types of tea:
- White tea
- Herbal teas
- Green tea
- Black tea

White tea comes from the Camellia sinensis plant which is native to China and India. It is the least processed variety. Some research has shown that it may be an effective tea in fighting various forms of cancer due to its high levels of antioxidants. It is also good for your teeth as it contains high levels of fluoride, catechins, and tannins that can strengthen teeth, fight plaque, and make them more resistant to acid and sugar.

Herbal teas are very similar to white teas but contain a blend of herbs, spices, fruits, and other plants in addition to tea leaves. Interestingly peppermint tea contains menthol, which can soothe the stomach and some think it helps with Irritable Bowel Syndrome (IBS).

Green tea originates from China, where late leaves are processed with heat using pan-firing or roasting – in Japan, the leaves are more commonly steamed. Green tea is high in flavonoids that can boost heart health by lowering "bad" LDL cholesterol and reducing blood clotting. Studies have shown that this type of tea can help lower blood pressure, triglycerides, and total cholesterol.

Black tea is made from the leaves of the Camellia sinensis plant, which is also the source of green and white tea. In this case, the leaves are dried and fermented, giving the tea its black colour and rich flavour. Black tea contains flavonoids which combat inflammation and help immune function. More studies have been done on green tea than black tea. Both are good in various respects and black tea seems to have caught up but basically, the jury is still out.

RED CABBAGE

Red cabbage is not particularly popular but has four times more antioxidants than regular cabbage. It contains anthocyanins which help the heart. It also has a high concentration of vitamins A and C – the former helping with vision.

BEETROOT AND BEET JUICE

My research has led me to find out that beetroot and beet juice are superfoods, so I now have half a cooked beetroot most days with two scrambled eggs on toast. There are five reported benefits.

1. Beetroots are packed with antioxidants and nitrates, and the latter cause the blood vessels to relax and so increases blood flow.
2. They are rich in beta-lactams which fight inflammation – and remember, chronic inflammation is associated with heart disease, cancer, and obesity.
3. Beetroot, with its antioxidants, reduces the damage to the cells caused by free radicals. Free radicals are associated with such conditions as Alzheimer's Disease, cancer, arthritis, and diabetes.
4. Beetroots reduce blood sugar after the meal so with that action, it is worth adding beetroot to your diet.
5. Beetroot has a high fibre content and helps you lose weight because the fibre gives satiety (a sense of fullness).

SPINACH AND KALE

Spinach is not very popular as it is not so pleasant to eat. It has a lot of antioxidants lutein and Zeaxanthin and these have a direct impact on blood vessels. It has been said they can help retinal degeneration, such as senile macular degeneration, but I think more evidence is needed.

Kale contains vitamin C and antioxidants Quercetin and Kaempferol, which are very potent in their
effect against free radicals. They are said to stop inflammation and protect the heart.

CHAPTER 14
SLEEP AND STRESS REDUCTION

Most people do not realise the importance of sleep, ideally having a regular sleep pattern. One should go to bed and wake up at the same time daily. The main function of sleep is the restoration of brain energy, switching off external impulses, and off-line processing of information acquired whilst awake. In other words, the brain is like a mini-computer. Sleep is involved in cerebral changes that are responsible for learning and memory consolidation. These functions are critical for brain development, physical and mental health, and maintaining cognitive function.

At the anecdotal level, I remember in school learning complex material in the evening, such as learning things word for word and going through this just before sleep. In the morning I would remember them word perfect. In other words, the brain-computer had been working overtime overnight!

INSOMNIA
Good sleep is important for general health and inadequate sleep (insomnia) in the long term will affect both short-

term and long-term memory. Lack of sleep can make us feel physically unwell – feeling sleepy, anxious, irritable, and unable to concentrate. In the long term, it is linked to heart disease, obesity, diabetes, premature ageing, and even road traffic accidents! There was a study in the US where mice were kept awake for two weeks – interestingly they developed diabetes mellitus. Some conditions are associated with sleep disorders:
- Narcolepsy
- Sleep apnoea

Narcolepsy is a specific condition of falling asleep suddenly at inappropriate times. The individual may feel drowsy and suddenly fall asleep while walking, talking, or driving. It is certainly rare and such a person is usually under a physician.

Sleep apnoea is when breathing stops. Often the individual makes loud or gasping/choking noises. Such individuals often have chronic obstructive pulmonary disease (COPD) and are obese – and are usually under the care of their doctor.

Other causes of sleep problems are:
- Physical/mental health issues
- Change in noise level or temperature of the bedroom
- Too much coffee/alcohol
- Watching television/using the internet late at night
- Shift work

Regarding mental health issues, anxiety is associated with brain overactivity and difficulty getting off to sleep. Depression is often associated with a broken sleep pattern or early morning awakening.

GOOD SLEEP AND DURATION OF SLEEP

If you are healthy you should have a fairly constant body time clock (circadian rhythm), with regular waking up time and time when you go to bed. Adults get sleepy well before midnight – and at that time, melatonin is released into the body. We should aim for between seven and nine hours of sleep each night – and I think ideally eight hours. I myself am usually asleep at 10.30pm and awake at 7.45am so I am getting 9.25 hours' sleep at night.

I have heard some people brag that they can manage on six hours of sleep. Many years ago I well remember when Margaret Thatcher was Prime Minister and she said she could manage on four hours of sleep. She seemed very proud of the fact, virtually bragging about it! It subsequently crossed my mind that having years of poor sleep may well have contributed to her dementia in her twilight years.

SLEEP CENTRE AND CIRCADIAN RHYTHM

For many years, going back to the time when I was a medical student, it was thought that the brain had a sleep centre in the hypothalamus – a small peanut-sized structure within the brain. To be precise it was thought that the supra-chiasmic nucleus (SCN) of the hypothalamus was involved. Later it was thought the "sleep centre" was in the hypothalamus and as a medical student, I was taught that melatonin is the hormone for regulation and the "wakefulness" centre was in the brain stem. Later still, it was thought the situation is far more complex, with wakefulness being regulated by a whole network of structures in the brainstem, hypothalamus, and basal forebrain – and is not sited in one part of the brain. A whole cocktail of neurotransmitters are involved during wakefulness and sleep and they include histamine, dopamine, norepinephrine, serotonin, glutamine, and acetylcholine.

As a medical student, I was taught that melatonin was the hormone for regulating the sleep-wake cycle. It was stated that darkness prompted the production of melatonin while light caused the production to stop – and so this synchronised sleep and wakefulness. A 1997 study in the Journal of Biological Rhythm noted that intense exercise in the evening boosted melatonin secretion by about 50%. Therefore, it is thought that vigorous exercise before sleep helps.

More recently, some US scientists have stated that SORT1 and NAD are raised in the morning and down in the evening – and this is what gets the body to sleep. This then allegedly turns on a gene called BML which is thought to control the circadian rhythm. This tells the liver and the brain to "calm down". I am not an expert in the field and the mechanism is more complex than we thought.

HOW TO ACHIEVE A GOOD CIRCADIAN RHYTHM

Poor sleep habits are not to be encouraged. This may occur because of a poor sleep schedule (eg., due to work demands) but it may be self-induced by waking late at night, drinking late at night, watching too much late-night television, etc. Late-night partying can also be a factor! It is important to have comfortable bedtime arrangements, with the exclusion of light (i.e. drawn curtains or blinds) as this can affect the melatonin level.

If there is a problem with the circadian rhythm (and of course, work arrangements may be unavoidable), then there are some tips to remember:

- Try to keep a regular sleeping regime
- Get regular daily exercise
- Sleep environment should be good – curtains/blinds to give darkness, adequate temperature, good mattress, etc. If there are financial constraints regarding heating, consider an electric blanket.
- Avoid coffee (caffeine) and alcohol before bed, and avoid smoking (nicotine)
- Just before sleep, it is advisable to avoid television or looking at the internet as these act as brain stimulants.
- Sex can induce sleepiness
- If you wake up worried about something write it down on paper, go back to sleep and deal with it in the morning.

CHANGES IN CIRCADIAN RHYTHM

Sometimes the circadian rhythm changes because of lifestyle – such as working overnight or variable shifts with erratic hours. Some people have a lifestyle that encourages late night hours and others may have to get up early in the morning. The circadian rhythm can also be affected by long-haul flights.

Jet lag occurs when you travel through several time

zones and your body clock is still at your point of origin. The body needs to adjust to the new time and when you arrive at the destination you may feel tired during the day. It can take some people a day or a few days to adjust to the new time.

As an anecdote, I remember going to Australia many years ago and having a connection in Singapore. I walked round that airport and decided I would sleep from Singapore to Melbourne. This was a good move as on arrival I was bright and alert and ready for the day ahead. In other words, I had put my sleep pattern on to Australia time.

DOES CORTISOL AFFECT SLEEP?

Cortisol has a particular circadian rhythm that affects sleep. In a healthy individual, the cortisol is high in the morning and lowest in the evening. If the body has chronic stress, as in an anxiety state, the body is in a constant high state of cortisol production. So to keep the cortisol level lower in the evening, you need to have light exposure during the day and do some exercise. Research has shown that regular physical activity at moderate intensity benefits people with chronic insomnia. Daytime workouts reduce the time you take to fall asleep and reduce middle-of-the-night awakenings (sleep fragmentation). The take-home message is high cortisol relates to poor sleep and exercise is an effective stress management technique to help your sleep pattern.

NIGHT OWLS AND INCREASED RISK OF DIABETES

I decided to review some papers on this topic and I wondered if I sleep at 11pm, am I considered a night owl? The answer to that is "no". It is referring to someone who tends to be awake late into the night. If you are a night owl you may do your homework at midnight and prefer to sleep late into the morning.

If you are a night owl you increase your risk of diabetes, based on a study at Brigham and Women's Hospital, Boston, Massachusetts. A person's preferred timing for sleeping is referred to as chronotype, and this is partly genetically determined so it may be difficult to change this. It is considered that having an evening chronotype is associated with a 19% increased risk of diabetes. Research from that hospital has previously found that those with evening chronotypes are more likely to have irregular sleep patterns and this puts them at higher risk of developing diabetes and heart disease.

A paper from that hospital was published in Annals Internal Medicine (2023) (S. Kianersi, Tianyi Huang) and looked at data from over 63,000 nurses, including whether they saw themselves as morning or evening people and also looked at diet, weight, drinking, and smoking. Around one in nine (just under 10%) were "evening people", just over a third stated they were "morning people", and the rest were "intermediate". An "evening person" (evening chronotype) had a 72% increased risk of diabetes but analysis of their lifestyle alone gave them a 17% increase of diabetes. Interestingly among those with the healthiest lifestyle, only 25% were "evening people". It was noted that night owls are more likely to drink more (sometimes retiring to late bars), smoke, have a poor diet, sleep less, and have unhealthy weight and poor physical activity.

It appears, therefore, that sleep timing is important but more important is lifestyle. Apparently those who worked day shifts and were night owls had an increased risk of diabetes, but night owls who worked overnight shifts did not. The hidden analysis relating to those two groups might be quite simple – the former group had inadequate sleep per 24 hours and the latter group had eight hours of proper sleep in the daytime. So this might be an area of interest, where personalised work scheduling is considered by employers.

STRESS REDUCTION

It is very important to avoid stress and in terms of stress management, it is important to relax and have a good sleep pattern. The majority of people do not realise the importance of sleep. One should set aside time to relax, whether reading newspapers, watching a film, or congenial conversation over a pint in a pub. From a general viewpoint, stress can reduce telomere length (see Genetics section) and shorten lifespan.

Stress is certainly a factor in many health problems and can precipitate heart problems – cardiovascular disease being the number one cause of death globally. Dr Harvanek of Yale did a study in 2021 which found that stress contributed to ageing outside of its impact on disease. He reported that control of emotion can defend us from the mental and physical effects of stress.

Avoiding stress is very important – and one should note that high-stress levels can contribute to cognitive decline in ageing adults. Chronic stress can increase your risk of mental and physical health problems like high blood pressure, sleep problems, and depression.

CHAPTER 15
EXERCISE AND WALKING

Exercise is important to keep our cells healthy and prevent ageing. Professor David Sinclair, the eminent geneticist at Harvard, has expressed the view: "It helps clear out the cellular garbage and keeps our cells functioning maximally." This process of cleaning up and regeneration is referred to as autophagy.

Interestingly Spermidine has an important role in inducing autophagy – which not only keeps cells healthy but also promotes longevity. Spermidine, according to the literature, is found in cheese, legumes, mushrooms, and soy. It is associated with a reduced risk of neurodegeneration, cardiovascular disease, and cancer-induced death in humans.

Keeping active is important, whether standing, walking, running, high-intensity training (HIIT), or playing football. Ideally, one should increase the heart rate and have some sweating.

PROLONGED SITTING

Sitting for prolonged periods, for example, eight hours at work or a prolonged journey in a vehicle is very disadvantageous. Time in front of the television for long periods is not good for the body. My maxim, or take-home message, is, "Keep on the move throughout life". This even includes the time when you are elderly.

Sitting for long periods increases the risk of heart disease, cancer, and depression. The American Journal of Epidemiology has reported that someone who sits more than six hours a day has an 18% increased risk of dying from heart disease and a 7.8% increased chance of diabetes compared with someone who sits for three hours a day.

What is the mechanism? Sitting for a long period causes the body to shut down at the metabolic level. When the muscles, particularly the leg muscles, are immobile the circulation slows. At the same time, you use less blood sugar and metabolise less fat – so by these two mechanisms, it is not surprising there is an increased risk of heart disease and diabetes.

Another rather complex mechanism is that with sitting there is a part to play by a gene called lipid phosphate phosphatase (LPP-1). This helps prevent blood clotting and inflammation to keep the cardiovascular system healthy but is significantly suppressed when you sit for a few hours.

CANCER RISK. The American Institute for Cancer Research has linked prolonged sitting with both breast and colorectal cancer. Dr Neville Owen at Baker Heart and Disease Institute, Melbourne, Australia, has indicated that sitting time is emerging as a strong candidate for being a cancer risk in its own right. Also, there is emerging evidence that suggests the longer you sit, the higher the risk. It seems that exercising will not compensate for too much sitting.

Alberta Health Services Cancer Care in Canada reports inactivity is related in Alberta to 49,000 cases of breast cancer, 43,000 cases of colon cancer, 37,200 cases of lung cancer, and 30,600 cases of prostate cancer per year.

DEPRESSION is also related to prolonged sitting and the mechanism postulated is that this reduces the circulation and less "feel good hormones" reach the brain. These are dopamine, serotonin, endorphins, and oxytocin and under normal circumstances, on reaching the brain they improve mood. One survey of 30,000 women found that those who sit for nine or more hours per day are more likely to be depressed than those who sit for six hours. Apart from the increased risk of cardiovascular disease, diabetes, cancer, and depression, we should also recall that prolonged periods of immobility can cause back pain, due to increased stress.

HOW LONG DO WE USUALLY SIT? According to the International Journal of Behavioural Nutrition and Physical Activity, people spend on average 64 hours a week sitting – i.e. about nine hours a day. I found this difficult to believe until I realised an office worker may have seven hours out of eight at a desk, travel sitting in a bus/car/train, come home, eat an evening meal, and then chat sitting on a settee or watching television. You may have some evenings which are very active and might go for a run, but this does not compensate for the prolonged immobility. It is worth remembering that with standing you lower the risk of heart disease, lower blood sugar levels, and have less stress and fatigue.

TAKE HOME MESSAGE. Prolonged sitting is clearly an adverse factor for health and it has been recommended that the maximum sitting time should be 30 minutes. So a common sense approach would be:
- Get up from the desk and walk around for five minutes every half an hour
- Soleus muscle calf exercises – having a session of raising and lowering the heel (soleus muscle push-up)
- some even consider fidgeting at a desk beneficial!

SOLEUS MUSCLE EXERCISE. As a medical student, I was aware that the soleus muscle is in the calf and is the primary muscle for standing, walking, and running. In relation to gym activities, I have learned of movements to strengthen the soleus muscle but had not heard about doing the exercises at a desk, until I read a particular paper recently. I am referring to a paper by Marc Hamilton, PhD, at the University of Houston, who studied the muscle carefully in the laboratory. He looked at the anatomical and cellular properties that make that muscle special. If you activate that muscle you will use more energy than normal. Hamilton looked at the soleus muscle push-up – with the heel raise and soleus contraction, the motor neurones were intensely activated (shown on electromyogram EMG). This is different to walking when the muscle is turned off once the heel starts to rise. What is particularly interesting is that he found people can lower blood glucose by 10% with a single session of soleus contraction – and this magnitude of response rivals that of hours of exercise. Instead of using intra-muscular glycogen, which is the stored carbohydrate in muscles, they are able to use fuel from the blood – i.e. blood glucose and blood lipoproteins. With these exercises you need to raise the calf, going on tiptoes, and you need to straighten the ankle in a fluid smooth motion. Ideally, you would do 60 exercises on the left and 60 on the right in a given session.

WALKING

Walking is well-known to have many health benefits, which I will shortly list and discuss. But firstly how many steps should you do per day? Ideally, you should do 10,000 steps (about five miles) and you may decide to find out how many you do using an app on Android or iPhone, but remember you need internet reception. An alternative is to buy a pedometer. In both the UK and the US, the number of steps taken is 3,000–4,000 steps per day (roughly 1.5 to 2 miles). The UK figure was provided by the NHS.

Young children and young adults do more. The International Journal of Behavioural Nutrition and Physical Activity indicates that young male children do between 12,000 and 16,000 steps per day and female children do between 10,000 and 13,000 steps per day. So older children and teenagers should aim for close to 12,000 per day.

The elderly and those with chronic conditions cannot reach the desired number. Adults aged 65 and older need 30 minutes per day five days a week – and the 30 mins might be divided into three sessions of 10 minutes. An alternative is 75 mins in a week with vigorous intensity, such as jogging, running, or hiking. I myself do countless sessions of 10 minutes in the garden!

A study in JAMA Internal Medicine found that older females who did 4,400–7,500 steps per day experienced a lower risk of all-cause mortality than people who did 2,700 steps per day. A 2020 study found that participants who took 8,000 steps per day had a 51% lower risk of dying by any cause compared to those who took 4,000 steps per day.

HEALTH BENEFITS OF WALKING
- Correction of obesity
- Lowers blood pressure (in the long term)
- Lowers risk of coronary artery disease
- Blood sugar improvement/reduces the risk of type 2 diabetes
- Improved muscle strength
- Improved balance
- Reduces knee and back pain
- Improves mental health/anxiety/depression
- Improves sleep

CORRECTION OF OBESITY
Regular walking helps to maintain a healthy body weight and lower fat. Interestingly research has shown that adults with excess weight are more likely to be depressed. Basically, they have poor self-image and have a 55% higher risk of developing depression compared with a person of normal weight. To combat obesity it is recommended that you do 30 minutes of moderate intensity, such as brisk walking, three times a week. These walks do not have to be done in one go but can be done in 10-minute sessions.

LOWERS BLOOD PRESSURE

Research by Lee IM et al, Medicine & Science in Sport and Exercise 40(7 Suppl) s512, showed that regular walking may improve both systolic and diastolic blood pressure. You need to remember that high blood pressure puts you at risk of heart disease, stroke, and kidney disease – so you should do everything you can to keep it controlled. Clearly, both medication and walking are important.

LOWERS RISK OF CORONARY HEART DISEASE

Research by Zhang H et al in the European Journal of Epidemiology 24, (4) 181-192 (published in 2009), has shown that 30 minutes of walking per day reduces the risk of coronary heart disease by 19%. Another paper by Lian X et al in Preventative Medicine 58, 64-69 (published in 2014) showed that walking 30 minutes at least five days a week decreased bad cholesterol (LDL) and increased good cholesterol (HDL).

So, the cardiac benefits from walking are well described and you can increase the benefit by the following:
- Walking briskly for sustained periods
- Focus on objects in the distance, as this can increase walking speed by 23%
- Climbing stairs and avoiding lifts/escalators
- As an exercise, you might step up and down on a stool, or use the first step on your stairs
- Some people do Nordic walking with poles

The usual walking speed is about three miles per hour but if your earphones are plugged into high-tempo music or pop hits you will find your walking speed increases to anywhere up to five miles per hour.

BLOOD SUGAR IMPROVEMENT/ REDUCED RISK OF TYPE 2 DIABETES

Regular walking may help improve blood sugar control and one study (Hamasaki 2016) showed that walking 30 minutes per day decreases the risk of type 2 diabetes by approximately 50%.

A 2013 study showed that walking 15 minutes after a meal helps stabilise the blood sugar. The mechanism is that with walking, the heart is pumping harder and the muscles are more active, so blood sugar is lowered and insulin increased.

IMPROVED MUSCLE STRENGTH

Muscle strength naturally declines with age unless there are preventative measures. I suggest you read up on gym-type exercises to do in your own home. In relation to walking, The Arthritis Foundation in the US states that walking can improve muscle strength and it can help flexibility and stamina. For the latter, more intense forms of walking may be helpful. For example, walking uphill activates three times more muscle fibres than when walking on the flat. So walking uphill gives an added benefit.

IMPROVED BALANCE
Walking will help people with their strength and balance. This is very important and you can reduce your risk of falling in old age, which can cause bone fractures and other injuries.

REDUCED KNEE AND BACK PAIN
Osteoarthritis and associated knee pain can cause walking difficulties. Interestingly research suggests that walking regularly may protect against the symptoms. My take is that perhaps increased strength in the surrounding muscles enhances joint stability.

Walking may also relieve back pain and was well described in a paper by Sitthiponvorakul (2018) entitled "Movement is certainly needed to keep the spine healthy: muscles around the spine need to be used". In this regard, do spine stretch exercises each morning, including touching your toes. I recently read an article that the deceased Duke of Edinburgh used to do certain exercises each morning, including touching his toes, and I gather King Charles has decided to follow suit with that activity!

BOOSTS MOOD
Walking boosts mood and reduces anxiety and depression (Shaman 2006). The mechanism is that regular walking enhances the release of endorphins, which stimulate relaxation and improve mood. The endorphins then interact with the brain receptors to give feelings of well-being. So with walking, there is:

- Improved mood
- Decreased anxiety
- Decreased depression

It is known that high-intensity exercise can produce a natural high, due to the release of endorphins. It is thought that low-intensity exercise over a prolonged period can increase the release of growth factor, which is said to increase the size of the hippocampus (a small structure near the pituitary). It is said to be small in those with anxiety and depression and can increase in size with low-intensity exercise.

IMPROVED SLEEP

Walking and other aerobic exercises increase the amount of deep sleep, which allows the brain to rest and recuperate. Dr Grimaldo of the Johns Hopkins Centre for Sleep and Wellness has reported that there is strong evidence that exercise helps you to fall asleep more quickly and improves sleep quality. Many parents want their young children to be really active late afternoon so that when they go to bed they are exhausted and soon fall asleep.

Interestingly Benson AN et al wrote a paper in Sleep Health 5(5) 487-494, which reported that people who took more steps throughout the day had better quality sleep than on the days where they were less active.

ACUTE EXERCISE AND RISE IN BLOOD PRESSURE

I thought I should write a paragraph on this as an anecdote. Normally blood pressure rises during exercise, due to increased cardiac output and increased uptake in the working muscles. There is an immediate increase in sympathetic activity which increases the heart rate and cardiac output. This therefore increases the stroke volume (increased output from the heart) and there is vasodilatation in the arteries of the skeletal muscle to accept the increased flow.

I am writing this to explain when your general practitioner or nurse sees you they need you in a resting or relaxed state to give a true reading.

CHAPTER 16

DRINKING WATER

Get into the habit of hydrating yourself as soon as you wake up. You tend to dehydrate whilst sleeping so ideally you should have 500ml–1 litre as soon as you go to the bathroom. Remember the body is mainly made up of water. The minimum amount of water a person needs to avoid dehydration is four to six cups per day. Instead of pure water, you might take tea, coffee, or orange juice – but the amount of fluids is important. Runners need to be sure they get enough fluid – marathon runners often have water provided at certain points.

In relation to drinking water, I would like to discuss three topics:
- Effect on the bowel
- Stroke prevention
- Reduction of cardiovascular risk

EFFECT ON BOWEL

Drinking water on an empty stomach helps in cleansing the bowel – by increasing bowel movement. If a person is prone to constipation the effect of water in the morning may solve the problem, by increasing peristalsis (contraction waves), encouraging evacuation and regulating bowel movement. At the personal level, I used to suffer intermittent constipation and found that taking 500ml–1 litre of water first thing in the morning solved the problem.

STROKE PREVENTION

It has been stated that drinking four to six cups of water may not only protect from strokes but improve a person's outcome in the event of a stroke. Researchers into strokes have found several preventable factors (uncontrolled hypertension/diabetes/raised cholesterol) but they also found that a number of patients come to hospital dehydrated. Loma Linda University in California is famous as a health services university and medical centre. They found that drinking at least five glasses of water per day is necessary for reducing stroke risk by 53%.

Research at the Johns Hopkins Hospital looked at the cardiovascular risk of dehydration and they found that patients who had not drunk enough fluid were nearly four times more likely to suffer worse outcomes after a stroke compared to those with normal hydration.

Research at the University of Arkansas showed that even mild dehydration in healthy young males could play a part in a person's cardiovascular risk (coronary artery disease and strokes). Interestingly they found the mechanism, which seems very logical. The effect of the dehydration was in the epithelium – the lining cells of blood vessels including the coronaries – and can affect the dilation and cause constriction.

CHAPTER 17
HIGH BLOOD GLUCOSE – DIABETES

Glucose in the body is used for fuel and a high blood sugar is known to accelerate ageing. Some glucose can be inadvertently attached to proteins – and then those proteins malfunction. So you need intermittent fasting to get rid of these glucuronidated proteins.

In the diagnosis of diabetes, you measure the glucose attached to Hb (HbA 1c) and this tells you roughly what level of glucose you have had in the body over the last month. It tells you if you are eating badly or if you are a type 2 diabetic. If there is an elevated HbA 1c then depending on the level you may be pre-diabetic or type 2 diabetic:

Pre-diabetes   5.7
Type 2 diabetes   6.5

A sub-optimal HbA1c is often reported as normal. In ascertaining the level it is important for the patient to have a good rapport with the GP, and if the test is done and you have not heard the result then you must contact the surgery. So many people are involved in the process that it is so easy for poor communication to occur. If there is a raised HbA C, whether in pre-diabetes or diabetes mellitus, the higher level of glucose makes the cell complacent and affects the repair systems. The sirtuins (discussed in the Genetics chapter) do not work so well as we age. If we keep glucose levels down at a young age we keep young. If blood glucose is higher we age more, as in diabetes. Patients given Metformin have a lowering of blood glucose and in general people on Metformin have less heart disease and cancer.

PRE-DIABETES

With pre-diabetes, there is a great danger of developing type 2 diabetes, and if that occurs then the ageing process is accelerated. As a medical student I was taught a lot about diabetes and its possible complications, and on the wards would see some very serious cases … e.g. with extensive gangrene of the foot or leg and often needing surgery. One was taught that you must try and stop pre-diabetes from becoming diabetes. The innuendo at that time was that if you have pre-diabetes then you have nothing to worry about but my view is that probably some adverse developments are starting at that stage.

In the US, they use risk models and do not get involved if a 5% risk for 10 years, and most risk models do not consider patients under the age of 40. Risk models are not used in the UK.

Relating to pre-diabetes, I think I should give an interesting story about a phone call from an old school pal. I naturally asked how he and his wife were keeping and he said they were fine, and then added he had recently gone suddenly blind in one eye but it soon recovered. One could say my antenna went up! Then he added quite proudly that he was pre-diabetic but not diabetic ... so he clearly thought everything was fine. He said his blood pressure was fine and gave me readings. With this history, there are several causes for his loss of sight but being pre-diabetic I would take the view that he might well have some vascular disease and the loss of vision of short duration was probably a transient ischaemic attack (TIA) i.e. "mini-stroke". I naturally passed some general comments and said he should liaise further with his general practitioner and I went on to say about an intermittent fasting regime and eating in a six-hour time frame. Sadly this fell on deaf ears and was told that was out of the question because his wife, being French, liked to have a big dinner. He seemed to have made no association between the TIA (probable) and the pre-diabetes.

I personally think the US Government is wrong to have screening at age 40, which is far too late. I suspect there are many pre-diabetics in their 20s, who may not even know they have the condition, and you must realise that pre-diabetes can occur at any age. I have a personal view that pre-diabetes should be screened for annually from the age of 25 and a reasonable number would be found. I would like to see the whole population screened annually and my view is that those found to have the diagnosis should start on Metformin. I say this because we know Metformin will lower blood glucose and stop organ damage in the pre-diabetic stage. It must not be used if kidney impairment is an issue as it could lead to lactic acidosis. Many will not agree with my thoughts on this, but when I have finished writing this book, I think I should convey my thoughts to NICE (National Association of Clinical Excellence) and let the experts deliberate. Remember new ideas do not always go down well ... and you will remember from earlier in the book how Jenner struggled to get acceptance for his vaccination programme!

CHAPTER 18

ULTRA-PROCESSED FOODS

Ultra-processed foods are a modern development and the term was introduced about 15 years ago. They are often high in salt and sugar and contain additives, emulsifiers, and preservatives. They typically lack fibre and nutrients and are unfortunately high in calories.

The consumption of these has greatly increased in recent years, both in the UK and Europe. Britain is in fact one of the world's biggest consumers of ultra-processed foods which account for more than half the calories eaten by the average adult and two-thirds of the average energy intake of children. At a recent Unicef UK Baby-Friendly Initiative Conference (2023) in Harrogate, Dr Van Tulieken, Associate Professor at University College London stated that there is a real crisis of industrialised processed foods being marketed to children. He is sure that these foods have addictive properties for both children and adults. He has also stated that poor diet has overtaken tobacco as the leading cause of death globally – and poor diet means an ultra-processed diet. Interestingly a study from the Institute for Health Metrics and Evaluation based in the US recently published in the Lancet (2023) stated that poor diet was responsible for 10.9 million deaths globally in 2017, compared with 8 million for tobacco.

WHAT ARE THE UNTRA-PROCESSED FOODS?

They include ready meals, frozen pizzas, shop-bought cakes, and potato-based snacks. However, many foods which are considered "healthy" are also ultra-processed, including supermarket sliced bread and "diet" foods and drinks. This is precisely the reason that I have stopped buying supermarket wholemeal sliced bread and now have "proper" baked bread which I have to cut, in the old-fashioned, traditional way!

SIGNIFICANT PROBLEMS

Many people, including Tim Spector of King's College London, think there are significant problems – and some conditions appear to be linked but the association is not finally proven. So possible considerations are:
- Possible increased cardiovascular disease
- Possible increased death rate
- Possible link to the development of tumours, particularly ovarian and brain
- Development of obesity

POSSIBLE INCREASE IN CARDIOVASCULAR DISEASE

A University of Paris study looked at 105,000 patients for five years and assessed their diet about twice per year. Those eating more processed food had more cardiovascular disease – 277 per 100,000 people compared with 142 per 100,000 in those eating less.

POSSIBLE INCREASE IN DEATH RATE

At the University of Navarra, Spain, a study of some 20,000 people was followed up for 10 years and their diet was looked at every two years There were 335 deaths during the study, but for those eating the least ultra-processed foods, there were 16 deaths.

POSSIBLE LINK TO DEVELOPMENT OF TUMOURS

A study from the Imperial College of Public Health (Lancet, Jan 2023) involved 200,000 adults and it is reported that the higher consumption of ultra-processed foods may be linked to the development of tumours, particularly ovarian and brain. I must emphasise the words **"may be linked"** but this is not proven. There may be other factors involved such as smoking, lack of exercise, or too much sugar in the diet.

DEVELOPMENT OF OBESITY

Obesity and being overweight are significant factors as far as longevity is concerned. Currently, more than 25% of children and 50% of the population are overweight.

The problem is that ultra-processed foods have little nutritional value. They also contain a lot of sugar which is unhealthy. Children tend to love the sweet taste and the soft texture. These foods contain little true natural food and without any fibre, they become a sort of slurry. With a lack of fibre, this food does not produce "satiety" and the children ask for more, thereby causing increased consumption of calories. Some authorities think that humans are not acclimatised to such foods and the hormones that tell your brain to stop eating have not evolved to cope with such modern foods. The crucial trigger factor is the lack of fibre and the effect on "satiety".

THE MICROBIOME

The "rubbish" food also has an effect on gut bacteria (the microbiome). This topic is discussed elsewhere but basically, thin people have higher counts of bacteroides (good bacteria) and overweight people have a much lower bacteroides count. The bacteroides are not good at absorbing fat so people with a high count absorb less fat and put on less weight. The microbiome microbes have an important part in regulating the immune system, which protects you from infections, and also in seeking and destroying cancers. Sometimes the microbiome is upset by antibiotics given to treat infections, and this sometimes leads to clostridium difficile diarrhoea.

There is evidence that the microbiome can have a major effect on how well we age. The Journal Nature has a paper from the Guangxi Academy of Science (China) where they looked at the microbes of 1,575 people, aged 20 to over 100. They found that the healthy centenarians had particularly high levels of bacteroides.

The US National Institute of Health has monitored in great detail what volunteers ate for a month. It was noted that subjects ate 500 calories per day more when given ultra-processed foods. This suggests the lack of fibre does not lead to "satiety", and therefore more is eaten.

Several studies since 2019 have shown when comparing normal unprocessed food and ultra-processed foods, those taking the ultra-processed take 17 calories per minute more than those on natural/unprocessed food.

Prof David Raubenheimer and Prof Steven Simpson of the University of Sydney are experts in nutritional energy. They have pointed out that ultra-processed foods can lead to reduced protein intake. We must remember that as we get older the need for protein rises so you need a good diet with plenty of protein coming from eggs, meat, fish, and beans. With this, you will have satiety, with less hunger and fewer cravings.

ULTRA-PROCESSED FOODS ARE ADDICTIVE

Research has shown that ultra-processed foods can be more addictive than class-A drugs. The fact is that ultra-processed food is not real food and has addictive properties. The lack of fibre in the food does not satisfy the brain and there is a problem with craving more, which is of course a feature of addiction. An analysis of 281 studies published in the BMJ (British Medical Journal) showed up to one in seven adults and one in eight children are believed to be hooked on ultra-processed foods.

Recently there was a young girl, probably early 20s, on

the television and she was grossly obese. She said she was going to have a new NHS drug at a cost of £2,500. This is taxpayers' money and I personally think that giving such a drug is morally and ethically wrong, and I cannot believe the learned professors on NICE have issued a permit for such medication. It is time they and the NHS got back to basics. There was no mention of what she was eating, but almost certainly she would be eating "rubbish" ultra-processed foods and then expect the general public to pay for her treatment!

OBESITY IN CHILDREN

This is becoming an increasing problem because of ultra-processed foods. The great problem is their bodies adapt to such a situation, with significant weight gain and indeed can lead to gross obesity. The great problem in these cases is that with the body's adaptation, the metabolism can be affected for years, and may actually lead to long-term obesity throughout life. This is very worrying precipitated by the parent's ignorance about the food they are giving to their children. Almost invariably they themselves are obese too, related to the overall family diet. The big worry is the close association of coronary artery disease, hypertension, stroke, reduced longevity, and deterioration in general health. It is worth noting that 25% of children are overweight and 50% of the population.

The take-home message is that such people should liaise with their general practice office and seek help, either from a doctor or maybe a Health Visitor.

UNPROCESSED FOODS.

I thought, for clarity, I should write a short paragraph on this. Unprocessed foods, or minimally processed, include fruit, vegetables, milk, meat, seeds, rice, and eggs. One caveat is that it is now thought red meat is not the most healthy and it is better to have white meat (chicken) or fish. To think in my childhood I lived on lamb chops and subsequently a steak maybe twice a week. But now, with the information available, I am on chicken or fish for my main meal.

PROCESSED FOODS

These have been altered to make them last longer or taste better – generally using salt, oil, sugar or fermentation. The category includes:
- Cheese
- Bacon
- Sausages
- Processed bread
- Tinned fruit and vegetables
- Smoked fish

At the personal level I used to have a full English breakfast and now I probably only have bacon rarely. I must admit I am partial to sausage and perhaps have that occasionally, about once per week!

CHAPTER 19
BENEFITS OF COFFEE

For years it was debated whether coffee was of benefit or not. It was noted to contain caffeine so it can cause insomnia. However, not everybody tolerates caffeine the same – some have no problem but others can get anxious and have insomnia and even physical dependence. Insomnia can usually be overcome by avoiding caffeine in the afternoon and evening. One report from Johns Hopkins University referred to some people having "caffeine-use disorder". Nowadays it is considered one of the best beverages and is observationally associated with better health. It is alleged that Britons drink 98 million cups of coffee per day!

There are many health benefits:
- Cardiovascular benefit
- Reduced incidence of carcinoma colon
- Performance-boosting effects
- May affect longevity
- Reduces risk of melanoma
- May reduce the risk of dementia

CARDIOVASCULAR BENEFITS

Observationally coffee drinking is associated with better health. The American College of Cardiology in the 71st Annual Scientific Session (2023) found that drinking two or three cups of coffee per day reduces the risk of heart disease and dangerous cardiac rhythm.

Now for some complex science. A crucial factor is that caffeine (in coffee) is a natural PCSK inhibitor which inactivates PCSK in the laboratory – and this leads to more receptors available to capture "nasty" LDL for metabolism and remove it from the blood. Since 2016 there have been PCSK inhibitor drugs (Alirocumab and Evolocumab) used together with statins in patients who require further lipid lowering. Interestingly there was a study in Glasgow in 2016 where there was intravascular ultrasound evidence of actual plaque regression in patients on PCSK9 inhibitors. In other words, PCSK inhibitors can get rid of nasty atheroma which is trying to block the coronary artery.

So with these comments about PCSK inhibitors and the fact that The American Journal of Cardiology reports that drinking two or three cups of coffee per day, there is pretty strong evidence to say we should drink coffee regularly.

REDUCED INCIDENCE OF CARCINOMA COLON.

Years ago I read a report that two cups of coffee per day reduced the incidence of carcinoma colon by 20%. I wondered whether the mechanism was increased peristalsis but I think the important fact is that the coffee bean is plant-based and contains significant soluble fibre. This ferments in the gut and feeds the good bacteria (the microbiome). We are learning more and more about bacterial health in the gut. Another fact worth recalling is that coffee beans are rich in polyphenols which are used by gut bacteria.

PERFORMANCE BOOSTING EFFECTS
These are well documented and include improved mental ability, and cognitive boosting effects and can be useful pre-workout.

MAY AFFECT LONGEVITY.
Longevity may be affected by increasing autophagy (described elsewhere).

REDUCES RISK OF MELANOMA
If one drinks regular coffee there is a 20% risk reduction for malignant melanoma (a malignant skin condition often related to excessive sun exposure).

MAY REDUCE THE RISK OF DEMENTIA
Prof Mariapino D'Onofrio et al of Verona University (2023) looked at the effects of espresso consumption on the brain, specifically focusing on its ability to counteract the formation of tau proteins. This new study found that compounds in espresso actively break down tau proteins. It is known that tau proteins accumulate in the brains of people suffering from degenerative diseases. The staff at

Verona University have suggested that drinking one cup of coffee per day could have a significant impact on reducing the incidence of dementia.

CHAPTER 20
BREAD

Bread overall is not a good thing. We all tend to eat some bread and I try and restrict myself to one to two slices per day. I must admit I used to have supermarket-seeded bread but have now changed to proper recently baked bread which one has to slice. I have looked at the packet and noted it is a superseed-grain loaf. I must say I have already noted the difference in texture: this should be more nutritious. Interestingly here in the UK, we buy 11 million loaves of bread per day.

Mass-produced bread is often stripped of nutrients and is packed with additives. In fact, in some cases, one slice contains more salt than some bags of crisps!

Bread is certainly high in carbohydrates and is fattening. This is why I restrict myself to two small slices of freshly baked bread – the slices being much smaller than those from the supermarket previously. This now brings me back to the time when I was doing regular outpatient medical clinics, dealing with all sorts of general medical issues – including diabetes, hypertension, and coronary artery disease. Often one would find that the patient is overweight, sometimes grossly so. Many doctors, with the pressure of work and the time factor, will keep to the main subject in question (such as diabetes or hypertension). Realising part of the underlying problem, and maybe the most significant underlying issue is their obesity, I would then raise the question of weight. This can be a very sensitive issue with a patient as they feel they are "all right" or take issue with any discussion about their weight.

Fortunately usually when I have raised the issue they are very grateful for the advice given. If the person was a long-distance lorry driver or taxi driver, for example, they would almost certainly say they had sandwiches for lunch. Bread would always seem to be the real enemy and I would explain about the calories taken. I sometimes used the analogy of "profit and loss on your bank account"… if you put more in the sum will go up, and food intake in relation to weight is the same.

CHAPTER 21
BANANAS, LEMONS, AND BROCCOLI

BANANAS

Bananas are certainly a very healthy food – and the important facts are that they are rich in fibre, potassium, and other minerals. I personally eat one or two at breakfast regularly and I think this reduces the possibility of certain diseases.

HIGH FIBRE in bananas is important and has been described as a pre-biotic food and a resistant starch to produce butyrate (butyric acid), which is one of the three main fatty acids in the gut. Healthy levels reduce abdominal discomfort in patients with Irritable Bowel Syndrome (IBS) and have been shown to improve digestion by reducing inflammation and helping intestinal function.

The effects of diet and gut microbiome (bowel bacteria) in gastrointestinal disease were carefully looked into at the University of Melbourne, Australia (G. Trachman, S. Fehily et al). It was noted that dietary factors in early life substantially affected bowel risk later in life. Exposure to ultra-processed foods in childhood and teens increased the risk of later development of inflammatory bowel disease

(Ulcerative Colitis and Crohn's Disease) and even colorectal cancer. The mechanism suggested was an alteration of gut flora (microbiome). Programmes such as Crohn's Disease Exclusion Diet were tried – i.e., removal of red meat and dairy products and replacement of higher fibre and plant food. For the fibre, bananas were recommended.

REDUCED RISK OF RENAL CARCINOMA. International Journal Cancer in January 2020 discussed fruits, vegetables and the risk of Renal Cell carcinoma. This was a prospective study of Swedish women – and it was noted that people who took bananas six times per week were 5% less likely to develop renal cancer.

HIGH IN POTASSIUM AND OTHER MINERALS. Being high in potassium helps lower blood pressure, which in turn reduces the risk of heart disease. Also, it might be added that if a person has heart disease, possibly with breathlessness due to some left heart failure or has oedema (swelling of legs) due to right heart failure, then it is highly probable they will be on diuretics ("water tablets"). These tend to lose potassium and the patient may be on potassium supplementation or take Spironolactone (with potassium retaining properties) or Amiloride. If, for whatever reason, the potassium becomes low then a banana may help keep the potassium in balance. If the potassium goes too low then heart irregularity may occur. So clearly if the patient has significant heart disease a banana will help the potassium, but would not be advised if the patient is already having potassium supplementation or is on a drug which retains potassium (Spironolactone, Amiloride).

HELPS SLEEP/BETTER BONES/POSSIBLY HELPFUL FOR VISION. Apart from potassium, bananas are rich in magnesium and contain some manganese. Magnesium is said to promote good quality restful sleep and a medium-sized banana gives 8% of the recommended daily intake of potassium. Manganese helps the body to absorb calcium and helps bone strength. Bananas also contain carotenoids which help with Vitamin A production that is needed for good eye vision.

LEMONS

REDUCE RISK OF HEART DISEASE AND STROKE. Lemons are certainly a good source of vitamin C and research has shown that eating fruit and vegetables rich in vitamin C reduces the risk of heart disease and stroke. It is worth recalling that the high level of vitamin C increases the antioxidant levels. Lemons are said to be rich in fibre but we do not eat them whole.

MAY PREVENT KIDNEY STONES as they contain citric acid which helps increase the urine volume and the pH (more acidic), which creates an environment less favourable for stone formation. Historically in my father's day, a popular remedy was Mist. Potassium Citrate and Hyoscamus – the potassium citrate acidifies the urine.

The caveat to the benefit is that lemon juice is so acidic that it can affect the mucosal lining of the oesophagus (which runs from mouth to stomach). It is well-known that acidic foods can contribute to gastro-oesophageal reflux (GORD) when food regurgitates upwards from the stomach. This can cause burning and discomfort. Incidentally, those who have the condition can find this affects sleep. It is important to sleep propped up and avoid stooping.

So given all the factors I do not take lemon – but would allow a very small amount to be squeezed on a piece of plaice!

BROCCOLI

Broccoli is high in many nutrients including fibre, Vitamin C, Vitamin K, iron, and potassium. It contains antioxidants … which I keep mentioning in this book! The antioxidants are lutein and zeaxanthin, which may prevent oxidative stress. It also contains high levels of glucoraphanin, a compound which is converted into the potent antioxidant sulforaphane (SFN) during digestion.

Fahey et al way back in 1997 suggested broccoli may have anti-carcinogenic properties. The sulforaphane (mentioned above) has been shown in the laboratory to inhibit breast cancer stem cells, and some experts subsequently suggest it could act against prostate cancer, breast cancer, colon cancer, and bladder cancer. But don't build up your hopes. Though the data is encouraging, much more information is needed to substantiate the hypothesis.

CHAPTER 22
TURMERIC

Turmeric has been known in India for its medicinal properties for ages and is part of everyday diet. To increase its bioavailability, take it with some black pepper, so absorption is increased. Some say it is better absorbed with olive oil/coconut oil. It is heat sensitive so it is best taken on its own, not heated with the cooking of food. It is interesting to note that part of my regime is at breakfast time to drink 500–750 ml of water and then two tablespoonfuls of olive oil (antioxidant) with a third of a tumbler-sized glass of pure orange juice. I then pour some turmeric (about one to two teaspoonfuls) and a sprinkling of black pepper into half a tumblerful of pure orange juice. So it is by pure chance that I was taking olive oil before taking the turmeric – effectively doing the right thing!

So what scientific evidence do we have for its usage? It contains curcuminoids – curcumin is known to lower cholesterol – and it has antioxidant and anti-inflammatory properties. I have already said I am a fan of antioxidants. It contains lipopolysaccharide which is said to give it anti-viral and anti-bacterial properties. It contains large quantities of vitamins C, E, and K as well as large amounts of calcium, copper, iron, magnesium, and zinc. So by taking it daily, it prevents free radical damage and strengthens immunity. It must not be taken in excess.

HEART DISORDER. Curcumin with its antioxidant properties helps lower "bad" LDL cholesterol, a major factor in coronary heart disease, and may help the endothelial lining of blood vessels.

HELPS DIGESTION. It is said to be excellent in helping digestion. Some of the chemicals in turmeric encourage the gall bladder to produce more bile – helping the digestive system – and some say it reduces gas/bloating symptoms.

CANCER. Due to its antioxidant properties, it may help prevent cancer by managing oxidative stress in the body. There is some research that curcumin present in turmeric kills cancer cells and slows the development of new blood vessels in tumours.

ALZHEIMER'S DISEASE. Curcumin certainly helps with inflammation and oxidative damage, which can be linked to Alzheimer's Disease, and some think it may even lessen the risk.

ENHANCED MEMORY AND TREATS DEPRESSION. In a depressed patient, the brain makes less Brain-derived neutropenic factors (BDNF), a protein that helps one to learn and remember things. This causes the hippocampus (associated with memory) to shrink. One study has suggested curcumin can raise BDNF levels and potentially undo changes. It has been shown to reduce plaques in the brain.

CHAPTER 23
CONCLUSION

I hope you have enjoyed reading this book and found the comments helpful. I wanted to make it an easy read and get the message across with regard to what action you need to take. I apologise for occasionally going into very complex genetics, which may have been a bit difficult to understand. I felt that some scientific evidence must be given to back up the comments.

In writing this book I did a lot of research and came across some new material. I realised, of course, the horrendous devastation of wars and the effect on the population. At one point in school, I was taught about the French Revolution and the Napoleonic Wars, but nothing was said about Napoleon's campaigns causing such tremendous numbers of deaths, far greater than World War I and II combined. I was briefly made aware of the American Civil War and on visiting the various battle sites, I learned how much the war meant to the US population. What I did not realise, however, was the number of deaths – far greater than the total number they lost in both WWI and WW II. I have to admit that basically, I was taught about British and American history. I had heard about the

China Opium wars, but not in detail, and did not realise about the same time as the American Civil War there was civil unrest with millions of deaths ... greater than Napoleon Wars, American Civil War, and World War I and II combined.

The advances in medicine were particularly interesting. I knew about Jenner in his development of the smallpox vaccination, which was a major advance and I well recall the Jenner Statue in Gloucester Cathedral. The advent of Penicillin in the 1900s was a magnificent development and now we probably should wait for genetic modification to prevent disease in the near future. We already know about the gene predilection for carcinoma breast.

The main impetus of the book, however, is the analysis of factors which can affect longevity and health. The advice to stop smoking has been around for years and it is now well-documented that it reduces your lifespan by 10 years, but also makes you genetically older. It is clear that we need a good diet and intermittent fasting, plenty of antioxidants, sleep well, social contacts, avoid psychological stress, and exercise regularly, even if we have an office job. By that, I mean if you are stuck at a desk from 9am to 5pm, get up and walk intermittently such as walking about for five minutes every half an hour and maybe doing soleus calf muscle pump exercises.

If you follow the advice given, I hope I have given you some extra years, and healthy ones as well.

www.ingramcontent.com/pod-product-compliance
Lightning Source LLC
Chambersburg PA
CBHW071713020426
42333CB00017B/2254